MW00749043

Air-Fryer Cookbook for Beginners 2021

Beginner's Guide to Air Fryers

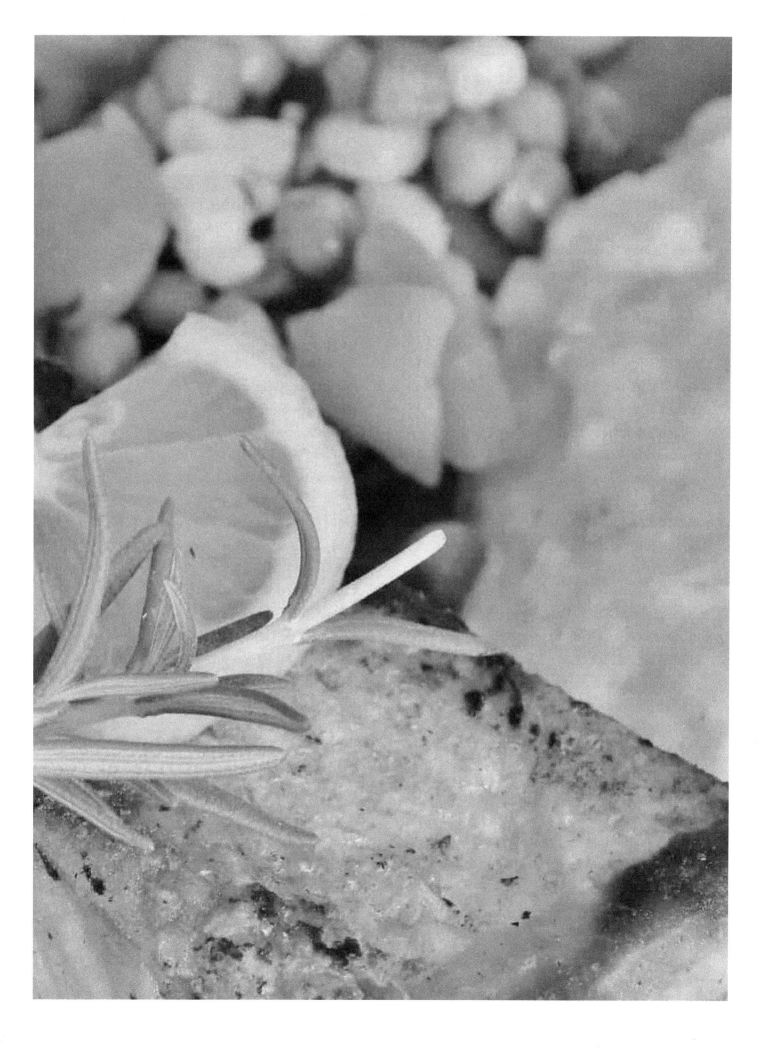

Table of Contents

Beginner's Guide to Air Fryers

Air fryers are quickly becoming a must-have in any modern kitchen. This easy-to-use appliance will save you time and money in the kitchen and maybe even a few extra calories! Looking to eat healthier? An air fryer can eliminate up to 50% of calories from fat while still making your food crispy and tasty!

Your new air fryer can be customized to cook anything from potatoes to fish! This handy guide will show you how to set up, use, and clean your air fryer so you will feel comfortable using it for many years to come! Many accessories are available for your air fryer that expand it's functions like pizza pans, skewer racks, and even cake barrels!

How Does an Air Fryer Work?

An air fryer uses the 'convection' method to circulate hot air around food that is placed in a tray or a basket. At a high speed, the outside of the food gets brown and crispy. This is called 'caramelization' which creates same effect as submerging food into hot oil. The air fryer works by coating the desired food in a thin layer of oil while circulating air heated up to 200 degrees C (392F). Your new air fryer can brown foods like potato chips, chicken, fish, steak, and even pastries using 70 to 80% less oil than a traditional deep fryer. Not everyone can have a full convection oven in their kitchen, but anyone can use an air fryer!

How to Set Up a New Air Fryer:

Your new air fryer features a power light, a timer, and a temperature gauge. Please refer to the formal instruction manual and diagram to learn about the symbols on the air fryer.

1. Remove the packing material and labels from the inside and outside of the air fryer.

2. Unlock the frying basket from the drawer and wash with hot, soapy water. Do not immerse your air fryer in water. Wipe with a clean, damp cloth and dry all parts thoroughly before first use.

3. Lock the clean basket into the drawer by sliding the handle between the notches on the top until it clicks. Now you are ready to cook!

Your new air fryer features a power light, a timer, and a temperature gauge. Please refer to the formal instruction manual and diagram to learn about the symbols on the air fryer.

Test Out Your Air Fryer:

Your air fryer is so easy to use once! Here is a step-by-step guide to frying!

1. Place your air fryer on a flat surface near an electrical outlet. Plug in and turn ON. Make sure there is at least 4" of air space around the entire fryer in order to adequately hot air and steam during use.

2. Open the fryer basket drawer and remove the inner basket. Place food inside the basket. Circulating air is what cooks the food, so be sure not to overfill the basket more than 2/3 full!

3. Return the fryer basket to the drawer and ensure it is fully locked in and the drawer is closed.

4. Select the desired temperature (between 175F and 400F).

5. If the air fryer is cold, add an additional 3 minutes to the specified cooking time for your food. Turn the dial to reflect that amount of time.

6. The HEAT light will illuminate.

7. In order to ensure even browning, open the fryer basket halfway during the cooking process and turn or shake the contents. Use oven mitts when handling the hot air fryer basket.

8. Keep cooking food at 5-minute increments until all pieces are fully cooked and uniformly browned.

9. Once the food has been cooked, allow 20 seconds for food to 'rest' before handling or removing from air fryer basket.

10. Turn off your air fryer by turning the timer dial to '0.' Unplug the air fryer when not in use.

Converting Recipes with Your Air Fryer

With a little know-how, you can enjoy your favorite food with half the fat caloriesusing your air fryer! Air fryers cook hotter than ovens, so a quick rule of thumb is to reduce the temperature on your air fryer by20 to 50 degrees and the cooking time by 20%. For packaged or frozen foods, the same rule applies. Just be sure to shake or turn the food halfway through the cooking pro- cess to be sure it's cooked thoroughly on the inside and evenly browned on the outside!

Helpful Tips forAir Fryer Success:

Thoroughly cleaning your air fryer after each use is the best way to ensure successful frying every time. But here are a few extra tips that will guarantee your appliance performs at its best!

1. Inspect the cords before each use. A frayed or damaged cord can cause serious injury.

2. Make sure there are no pieces of debris inside your air fryer before using it. If it's been a long time since you used your air fryer, inspect it for loose debris, dust or any other damage. If any of the components are damaged, contact the manufacturer for replacements.

3. Always use your air fryer on a level surface. This ensures proper cooking and a safe user experience.

Air Fryer:

Make sure your air fryer is completely cooled and clean before storing. Keep it in an upright position and make sure the cords are secure by gently tucking them into the drawer.

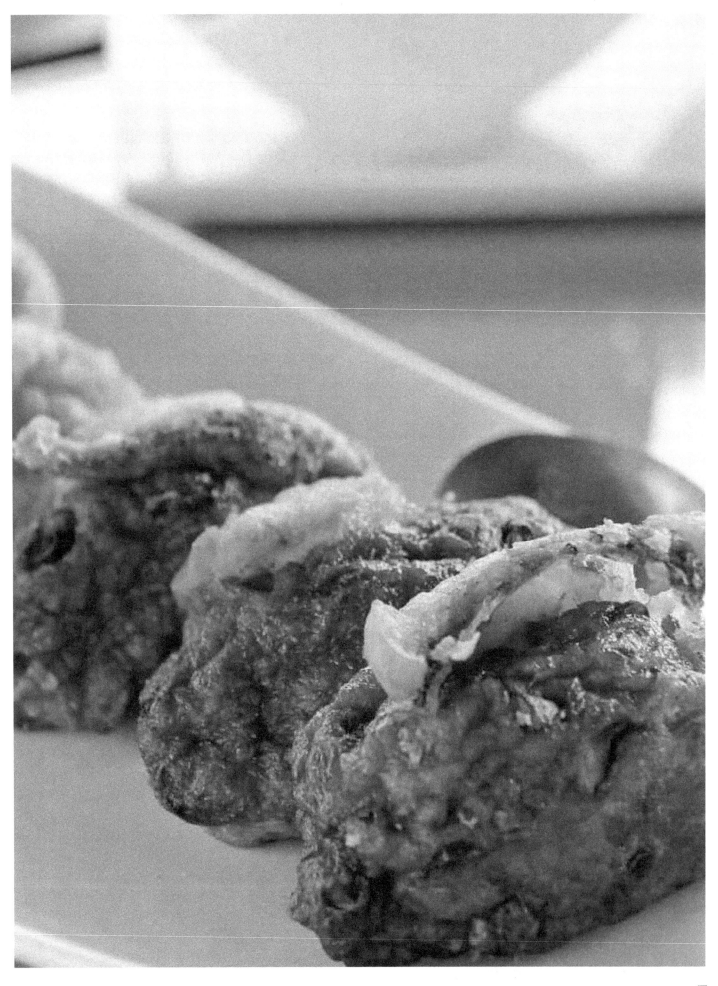

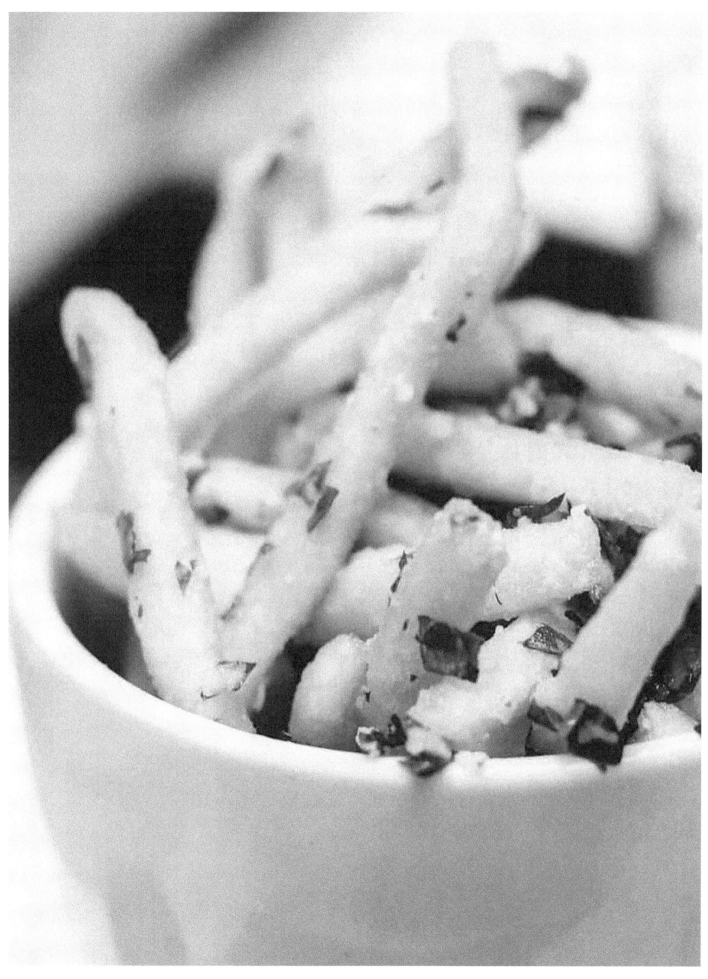

Chicken

Chicken Wings

Serving: 4　　**Cooking Time: 20 minutes**

Nutritional values

Calories 350 kcal

Fat 8.27 g

Total Carbs 14.89 g

Protein 50.46 g

Ingredients

2lb. chicken wings

1/2 cup BBQ sauce

1 tbsp soy sauce

1/4 tsp black pepper

For Garnishing:

1/2 cup cilantro, chopped

Directions:

1. Add all the ingredients to the chicken wings and let marinate for an hour.
2. Preheat the air fryer to 380F.
3. Transfer the chicken wings into the air fryer basket.
4. Cook for 20 minutes at 400F until crisp and lightly browned.
5. Transfer to a serving bowl, sprinkle chopped cilantro and serve.

Sticky Lemon Drumsticks

Serving: 3　　**Cooking Time: 15 minutes**

Nutritional values

Calories 783 kcal

Fat 40.02 g

Total Carbs 50.05 g

Protein 56.01 g

Ingredients

2lb. chicken drumsticks

1/2 cup honey

3 tbsp teriyaki sauce

2 tbsp butter

1 tbsp lemon juice

1 tbsp olive oil

For Garnishing:

1/2 cup parsley, finely chopped

Lemon wedges

Directions:

1. Preheat the air fryer to 360F.
2. Use an oil brush, to coat the drumsticks very lightly with olive oil.
3. Place the drumsticks in the air fryer basket.
4. Cook for 15 minutes, turning the drumsticks halfway after few minutes with a tong.
5. Meanwhile combine all the remaining ingredients to a bowl and microwave for 3 minutes.
6. When the drumsticks are cooked through, brush them with the prepared sauce until well coated.
7. Garnish with chopped parsley and serve hot with lemon wedges.

Tandoori Masala Chicken

Serving: 6   **Cooking Time: 25 minutes**

Nutritional values

Calories 311 kcal

Fat 8.89 g

Total Carbs 5.87 g

Protein 49.26 g

Ingredients

3 lb. chicken

2 cup yogurt

1 tbsp ginger

1 tbsp garlic paste

1 tsp turmeric

1 tsp red chili powder

1 tsp ground cumin

4 tbsp lemon juice

For Garnishing:

1 cup onion, sliced into rings

4-5 lemon wedges

Directions:

1. Start by preparing a marinade, in a large mixing bowl, combine yogurt, ginger garlic paste, turmeric, chili powder, cumin and lemon juice; mix until well combined.

2. Rinse the chicken and pat the excess moisture with paper towel.

3. With the help of a sharp knife, mark the slits in the center of each chicken.

4. Pour the marinade over the chicken and let marinate for 2 hours.

5. Line the air fryer basket with aluminum foil.

6. Preheat the air fryer to 360F.

7. Place the chicken into the basket and cook for 25 minutes at 380F.

8. Once the chicken is done, transfer the chicken to a serving dish.

9. Top with onion rings and serve with lemon wedges.

Rotisserie Chicken

Serving: 6   **Cooking Time: 30 minutes**

Nutritional values

Calories 392 kcal

Fat 12.99 g

Total Carbs 3.53 g

Protein 62.22 g

Ingredients

4 lb. whole chicken

2 tbsp olive oil

For Dry Rub:

1 tbsp garlic powder

1 tbsp onion powder

1 tbsp paprika

1 tbsp curry powder

Salt and pepper to taste

Directions:

1. Preheat the air fryer to 360F for 10 minutes.

2. Thoroughly wash the chicken, remove the neck and giblets.

3. Pat the excess moisture with paper towel.

4. With the help of a sharp knife, mark the slits in the middle of the chicken.

5. Brush the chicken with oil; set aside.

6. In a large mixing bowl, mix all the spices together.

7. Generously rub the spices onto each side of the chicken.

8. Place the chicken into the air fryer basket.

9. Cook at 400F for about 15 minutes.

10. Turn the chicken upside down and cook for another 15 minutes at 360F.

11. Once the chicken is done cooking, transfer it to a large serving dish.

12. Let rest for 10 minutes at room temperature, slice and serve.

Crispy Garlic Chicken with Lemon Dip

Serving: 6   **Cooking time: 20 minutes**

Nutritional values

Calories 384 kcal

Fat 14.7 g

Total Carbs 6.59 g

Protein 53.41 g

Ingredients

3lb. chicken

Coating:

1 cup bread crumbs

1 cup parmesan cheese

1 tbsp onion powder

1 tsp garlic powder

1 tbsp oil

2 eggs

For Lemon Dip:

1/4 cup sour cream

1 tbsp lemon juice

1/4 tsp paprika

Salt to taste

Directions:

For Lemon Dip:

1. Combine all the ingredients into a small serving bowl and set aside.

For Chicken:

2. Thoroughly wash the chicken, pat the excess moisture with paper towel.

3. In a large mixing bowl, combine bread crumbs, parmesan cheese, onion powder and garlic powder. In another bowl beat egg and oil until frothy.

4. Dip each chicken piece into the egg and then into the bread crumb mixture.

5. Preheat air fryer for few minutes at 380F.

6. Arrange the chicken into the basket, shaking off any excess bread crumbs.

7. Cook for 20 minutes.

8. Serve the chicken with lemon dip.

Chicken Nuggets

Serving: 8   **Cooking time: 15 minutes**

Nutritional values

Calories 228 kcal

Fat 11.8 g

Total Carbs 3.63 g

Protein 24.94 g

Ingredients

2lb. chicken breast, boneless and cut into 1/2 inch pieces

1 cup bread crumbs

1 large egg

2 tbsp Italian seasoning

1 tsp olive oil

Salt and pepper to taste

Directions:

1. Preheat air fryer to 400F for few minutes.

2. In a large mixing bowl, mix bread crumbs, Italian seasoning, salt and pepper.

3. Whisk the egg and olive oil in a medium bowl.

4. Dip chicken pieces in the egg mixture and then into the crumb mixture.

5. Place the chicken nuggets into the air fryer basket.

6. Be careful not to over crowd the basket. Try to cook in batches if needed.

7. Air fry for 15 minutes, turning halfway until nice golden and crispy.

Roasted Almond Chicken

Serving: 8 **Cooking time: 30 minutes**

Nutritional values

Calories 303 kcal

Fat 10.51 g

Total Carbs 2.53 g

Protein 46.4 g

Ingredients

4lb. whole chicken

1/2 cup almonds, coarsely chopped

3 tbsp Italian seasoning

1/4 cup lemon juice

3 tbsp butter

1/4 cup parsley, finely chopped

Salt to taste

Directions:

1. Clean and pat dry the chicken.

2. In a small mixing bowl, combine almonds, Italian seasoning, lemon juice, butter, parsley and salt; mix until well combined.

3. Generously rub the mixture all over the chicken.

4. Spray the air fry basket with cooking spray and preheat the air fryer to 400F.

5. Transfer the chicken to the basket and roast for 30 minutes flipping halfway through.

6. Serve with your favorite dip.

Chicken Pie

Serving: 6 **Cooking time: 20 minutes**

Nutritional values

Calories 635 kcal

Fat 39.62 g

Total Carbs 45.61 g

Protein 23.77 g

Ingredients

1lb. chicken breast, boneless	2 clove garlic, minced
1lb. or 1 package of puff pastry frozen	1/2 cup milk
1 small onion, chopped	1 tbsp Worcestershire sauce
1 cup carrot, diced	1 tbsp plain flour
1 cup peas	1 tbsp oil
1 cup potatoes, cubed	1 egg yolk
1 cup mushroom, sliced	Salt and black pepper to taste

Directions:

1. In a fry pan heat oil until shimmering.

2. Add onion and garlic, sauté for 5 minutes.

3. Add flour and cook for 30 seconds, immediately add milk, Worcestershire sauce and all the vegetables.

4. Season with salt and pepper.

5. Cook until the mixture starts to bubble.

6. Once thickened remove from heat; set aside.

7. On a lightly floured surface, roll the pastry dough out, about ¼ inch thick rectangle.

8. Using a round cookie cutter or a small glass, cut out circles.

9. Spoon a small amount of chicken filling into the centers of each circle.

10. Brush with the egg yolk around the perimeter of each circle.

11. Top with the second pastry cut out and seal the edges with a fork.

12. Brush the pies with egg yolk, poke 2-3 holes with the help of a fork.

13. Preheat the air fryer to 400F.

Chicken Sandwich

Serving: 6   **Cooking time: 25 minutes**

Nutritional values

Calories 165 kcal

Fat 10.8 g

Total Carbs 2.96 g

Protein 14.27 g

Ingredients

1lb. ground chicken

1/2 cup bread crumbs

1/4 cup onion, finely chopped

1/2 cup green bell pepper, chopped

2 clove garlic, minced

1 large egg

2 tbsp oil

Salt and black pepper to taste

For Sauce:

1/2 cup chili garlic sauce

1 tsp Dijon mustard

1/4 tsp black pepper

For Filling:

6 sandwich buns

1 head romaine lettuce, chopped

1 large tomato, sliced

Directions:

1. In a food processor mix ground chicken, bread crumbs, garlic, egg, oil, salt and black pepper. Process until well combined.

2. Transfer the mixture into a large mixing bowl, add onion and bell pepper; mix well.

3. Form the mixture into 1 inch thick, 6 oval patties.

4. Preheat the Air Fryer to 380F.

5. Place the chicken patties into the bottom of the Air Fryer.

6. Cook for 25 minutes, turning patties after 12 minutes with tong.

For Sauce:

7. In a small mixing bowl, mix all the sauce ingredients and set aside.

For Assembling:

8. Spread some sauce onto the bottom halves of the buns, top with a Pattie.

9. Place some lettuce and a sliced tomato and on top of the patties.

10. Sandwich with the second bun and serve.

Mexican Chicken Wrap

Serving: 8   **Cooking time: 15 minutes**

Nutritional values

FOR CHICKEN:

Calories 215 kcal

Fat 12.19 g

Total Carbs 1.04 g

Protein 23.73 g

FOR SOUR CREAM:

Calories 21 kcal

Fat 1.53 g

Total Carbs 1.32 g

Protein 0.55 g

Ingredients

2lb. chicken breast

1 tbsp vinegar

1 tbsp soy sauce

1 tbsp chili sauce

1 tsp black pepper

1 tbsp olive oil

Salt to taste

For Sour Cream:

1/2 cup sour cream

2 cloves garlic, minced

1 tsp lemon juice

1/2 tsp green chili, finely chopped

For Filling:

8 tortillas

1 cup carrot, shredded

1 cup cabbage, shredded

1 cup Lettuce, shredded

1/2 cup tomatoes, chopped

1 cup cheddar cheese, shredded

1 cup mozzarella cheese, shredded

Directions:

1. Marinade the chicken breast with vinegar, soy sauce, chili sauce, olive oil, black pepper and salt. Refrigerate and let marinate for an hour.

2. Preheat the air fryer to 400F.

3. Place the marinated breast into the air fryer basket and bake for 15 minutes, turning the chicken after few minutes with tong to make sure the chicken breast are evenly browned.

4. Once the chicken is done, transfer it to a large serving plate; slice and let cool at room temperature.

For Sour Cream:

5. Mix together all the ingredients and set aside.

For Assembling:

6. Place the sliced chicken down the center of each tortilla.

7. Add shredded carrot, cabbage, lettuce and chopped tomatoes.

8.

Thai Chicken Skewers

Serving: 12   **Cooking time: 20 minutes**

Nutritional values

Calories 246 kcal

Fat 14.95 g

Total Carbs 2.2 g

Protein 24.86 g

Ingredients

3lb. chicken breast, cubed

1/4 cup peanuts, crushed

2 cloves garlic, minced

4 tbsp coconut cream

1 tsp brown sugar

1 tbsp peanut sauce

1 tbsp fish sauce

1 tsp ground ginger

2 tbsp heavy cream

1/2 tsp red chili powder

1 tbsp lemon juice

12 wooden skewers

For Garnishing:

½ cup sesame seeds, optional

Lime wedges

Directions:

1. Start by preparing a marinade, except peanuts; blend all the ingredients together until well combined.

2. Place the cubed chicken into a large mixing bowl, pour the marinade and let marinate for 3-4 hours.

3. Thread the marinated chicken onto the skewers. Sprinkle crushed peanuts.

4. Spray the air fry basket with cooking spray and preheat at 380F for few minutes.

5. Carefully place the skewers into the air fryer basket and cook for 20 minutes.

6. Try not to over crowd the basket. Cook in batches if necessary.

7. Sprinkle sesame seeds and serve with lime wedges.

BBQ Chicken Pizza

Serving: 6   **Cooking time: 15 minutes**

Nutritional values

Calories 313 kcal

Fat 9.64 g

Total Carbs 25.88 g

Protein 29.65 g

Ingredients

1lb. chicken, boneless and cubed

3/4 cup BBQ sauce

For Filling:

1 package fresh pizza dough

1 cup pizza sauce

1 cup mozzarella cheese

1 cup cheddar cheese

¼ tsp chili flakes

Directions:

1. Marinate the chicken pieces with BBQ sauce.

2. Preheat air fryer to 400 F.

3. Divide the dough into 6 equal pieces.

4. On a lightly floured surface, roll the dough out, into 6-inch thick circles.

5. Spread pizza sauce on each circle.

6. Place the marinated chicken pieces on top of the sauce.

7. Top with some cheese and place it carefully into the air fryer basket.

8. Cook for 15 minutes at 360F.

9. Sprinkle some chili flakes and serve hot.

Chicken Lollipops

Serving: 4 **Cooking time: 30 minutes**

Nutritional values

Calories 373 kcal

Fat 22.55 g

Total Carbs 10.45 g

Protein 30.88 g

Ingredients

6 Chicken wings

For Marinade:

1 tbsp Worcestershire sauce

1 clove garlic, minced

1/2 tsp chili sauce

1 tsp black pepper

Salt to taste

For Batter:

1/4 cup flour

2 tbsp corn flour

1 large egg

Directions:

1. Preheat air fryer for few minutes.

2. Cut off the bone part and collect all the flesh at one end. Spray the wings with cooking spray and set aside.

3. Mix all the marinade ingredients to a large mixing bowl.

4. Place the prepared chicken lollipops in the marinade and let marinate for 1 hour.

For Batter:

5. In another large mixing bowl, mix all the batter ingredients until smooth and creamy.

6. Wrap the exposed bone part with a small piece of aluminum foil from avoiding dark and sticky.

7. Dip the meat end of each chicken into the batter and then immediately to the air fryer basket.

8. Cook at 360F for 30 minutes, flipping halfway through.

9. Once the chicken lollipops are nice golden and crispy.

10. Prior to serving remove the foil and serve with your favorite dip.

Almond Stuffed Chicken

Serving: 4 **Cooking time: 25 minutes**

Nutritional values

Calories 857 kcal

Fat 59.91 g

Total Carbs 4.37 g

Protein 72.88 g

Ingredients

4 chicken breast

1/4 cup almonds, roasted and chopped

1 cup cream cheese

1 cup cheddar cheese

1 clove garlic, minced

1 tbsp olive oil

Salt and pepper to taste

For Garnishing:

1/3 cup parsley, chopped

Lemon wedges

Directions:

1. Preheat air fryer to 400F.

2. With the help of sharp knife, mark the slits in the middle of each breast to form pockets.

3. Rub olive oil all over the chicken.

4. In a small mixing, combine cream cheese, cheddar cheese, almonds, garlic, salt and pepper.

5. Spoon the cheese mixture into each chicken pockets.

6. Secure the pockets with toothpicks.

7. Place the stuffed chicken into the air fryer basket and cook for 25 minutes.

8. Garnish with fresh parsley and lime wedges.

Turkey

Butter-Honey Glazed Turkey

Serving: 6　　**Cooking time: 20 minutes**

Nutritional values

Calories 670 kcal

Fat 18.97 g

Total Carbs 12.91 g

Protein 107.56 g

Ingredients

6lb. whole turkey

1/4 cup butter

1/4 cup honey

1 tsp rosemary

1 tsp thyme

1 tsp oregano

1 tsp paprika

1 tsp black pepper

2 tbsp olive oil

Salt to taste

Directions:

1. Preheat air fryer to 400F.
2. Brush the olive oil all over the turkey.
3. In a small bowl, combine butter, honey, rosemary, thyme, oregano, paprika, black pepper and salt; rub the mixture generously all over the turkey.
4. Place the turkey into the air fryer basket and cook for 20 minutes or until the final temperature of turkey reads 165F.
5. Flip the turkey upside down after 10 minutes.
6. Remove the turkey and let rest for 10 minutes before serving.

Pineapple Turkey Kabobs

Serving: 8　　**Cooking time: 30 minutes**

Nutritional values

Calories 283 kcal

Fat 18.24 g

Total Carbs 13.77 g

Protein 15.91 g

Ingredients

2lb. turkey, boneless & cubed

2 cups pineapple, diced

2 medium onion, cubed

1 cup green bell pepper, cubed

For Marinade:

1 cup pineapple juice

2 clove garlic, minced

1 tsp ginger

1 tbsp Worcestershire sauce

1 tbsp vinegar

Salt and black pepper to taste

8 wooden skewers

Directions:

1. Start by preparing a marinade; pour all the ingredients into a large mixing bowl.
2. Add turkey and marinate for 3 hours.
3. Spray the air fryer basket with some cooking spray and preheat at 400F.
4. Alternately thread turkey, pineapple, onion and bell pepper onto the skewers.
5. Place the skewers into the prepared basket and cook for about 30 minutes or until turkey temperature reaches 165F.

Lemon Garlic Turkey

Serving: 6   **Cooking time: 25 minutes**

Nutritional values

Calories 267 kcal

Fat 12.96 g

Total Carbs 2.47 g

Protein 33.47 g

Ingredients

2 lb. turkey breast, with skin

1 cup cherry tomatoes

2 clove garlic, minced

1/4 cup fresh lemon juice

2 tbsp lemon peel, grated

1 tsp oregano

1 tsp thyme

1 tbsp olive oil

Salt to taste

For Garnishing:

Lemon, sliced

Directions:

1. Thoroughly wash the turkey breast and pat the excess moisture with paper towel.

2. Grease the air fryer basket with olive oil and preheat at 360F.

3. In a small mixing bowl, mix garlic, lemon juice, lemon peel, oregano, thyme and salt.

4. Generously rub the mixture all over the turkey breast.

5. Place the turkey breast and cherry tomatoes into the prepared air fryer basket.

6. Cook for 25 minutes.

7. Garnish with some sliced lemon and serve hot.

Turkey Pattie with Avocado Salad

Serving: 8   **Cooking time: 20 minutes**

Nutritional values

Calories 302 kcal

Fat 26.49 g

Total Carbs 3.02 g

Protein 12.13 g

Ingredients

1 lb. ground turkey

1/2 cup breadcrumbs

1/2 cup green onion, chopped

1/2 cup onion, chopped

1 clove garlic, minced

1 large egg

1 tbsp teriyaki sauce

1 tsp oil

Salt and pepper to taste

For Avocado Salad:

1 large avocado, diced

1 cup cherry tomato

1/2 cup onion, chopped

Salt and black pepper to taste

Directions:

1. In a large mixing bowl mix all the ingredients together.

2. Shape the mixture into 8 patties, 1/2 inch thick.

3. Preheat the air fryer to 400F.

4. Place the patties into the air fryer basket and cook for 20 minutes.

5. Meanwhile mix all the salad ingredients to a serving bowl and set aside.

6. Serve the patties with avocado salad.

Mexican Turkey Tacos

Serving: 6 **Cooking time: 20 minutes**

Nutritional values

Calories 402 kcal

Fat 13.99 g

Total Carbs 35.61 g

Protein 34.43 g

Ingredients

1lb. ground turkey

1 tbsp taco seasoning

1/4 cup onion, finely chopped

1 tbsp lemon juice

1 tbsp olive oil

Salt to taste

For Filling:

12 corn taco shells

2 cup black beans

1 cup salsa

1 cup lettuce, shredded

2 cups mozzarella cheese

Directions:

1. In a large skillet, heat oil over medium-high heat, sauté onion for 5 minutes.
2. Add ground turkey, taco seasoning, salt and fry until nice golden brown.
3. Once the turkey is done, remove from heat.
4. Add lemon juice and set aside.
5. Spoon the turkey mixture into the taco shells.
6. Add black beans, salsa and mozzarella cheese.
7. Line the air fryer basket with aluminum foil, spray with some cooking spray and preheat at 400F for 8 minutes.
8. Place the tacos into the basket and cook for 10 minutes until crispy.
9. Transfer the tacos to a serving dish, top with lettuce and serve immediately.

Pistachio Stuffed Turkey Breast

Serving: 6 **Cooking time: 25 minutes**

Nutritional values

Calories 568 kcal

Fat 35.12 g

Total Carbs 7.88 g

Protein 54.48 g

Ingredients

3lbs. turkey breast

1/4 cup butter

1 cup pistachio, chopped

1/4 cup walnuts, chopped

1/2 cup apples, cubed

1 tbsp thyme

Salt and pepper to taste

Directions:

1. Preheat the air fryer to 400F.
2. Season turkey breast with butter, salt and pepper.
3. In a small mixing bowl, mix pistachio, walnuts, apples and thyme, toss until well mixed.
4. With the help of a sharp, mark slits in the center of each breast.
5. Stuff each turkey pockets with the pistachio filling.
6. Roll up each breast tightly and secure with toothpick.
7. Place the pockets into the air fryer and cook for about 25 minutes.
8. Once the turkey is done remove toothpicks and serve.

Turkey Quesadilla

Serving: 2   **Cooking time: 20 minutes**

Nutritional values

Calories 1391 kcal

Fat 61.81 g

Total Carbs 127.63 g

Protein 84.08 g

Ingredients

1lb. ground turkey

1/2 tsp dried oregano

1 can green chilies, chopped

2 clove garlic, minced

1 tbsp oil

1 tsp salt

For Filling:

4 tortillas

1 cup cheddar cheese

1 cup mozzarella cheese

1 cup corn

1 cup sweet red pepper

1 cup sweet yellow pepper

Directions:

1. In a large nonstick skillet over medium to high heat, heat oil, sauté garlic for 2 minutes.
2. Add turkey and cook until no longer pink.
3. Add green chilies, oregano and salt. Cook for 8 minutes.
4. Once the turkey is done, remove from heat.
5. Spray air fryer basket with cooking spray and preheat at 360F.
6. Place 1 tortilla on a cutting board.
7. Spread half of the turkey mixture in the center of each tortilla.
8. Top with corn, red pepper, yellow pepper, corn & cheese.
9. Place second tortilla over the top of the cheese.
10. Carefully place the Quesadilla into the prepared basket & cook for about 10 minutes or until golden & crispy.

Cranberry Turkey Wings

Serving: 4   **Cooking time: 15 minutes**

Nutritional values

Calories 774 kcal

Fat 42.29 g

Total Carbs 26.98 g

Protein 69.07 g

Ingredients

3lbs. Turkey wings

1/2 cup cranberry, dried

1/2 cup cranberry sauce

1/4 cup green onion, finely chopped

1 tsp smoked paprika

1 tsp black pepper

Salt to taste

Directions:

1. In a large mixing bowl, place the turkey wings; season with paprika, black pepper and salt.
2. Add the dried cranberry and sauce; rub the mixture over the wings and let marinate for 2 hours.
3. Preheat air fryer to 380F for 10 minutes.
4. Place the wings into the basket and cook for 15 minutes.
5. Once the wings are done, remove from the air fryer.
6. Garnish with green onion and serve.

Pulled Turkey Sandwich

Serving: 4 **Cooking time: 40 minutes**

Nutritional values

Calories 373 kcal

Fat 17.08 g

Total Carbs 1.78 g

Protein 49.78 g

Ingredients

2 lbs. Turkey breast

1 tbsp oyster sauce

1 tbsp Worcestershire sauce

1 tsp olive oil

1 tsp black pepper

Salt to taste

For Filling:

8 slices of bread, toasted or browned in pan

Cheddar cheese, slices

1 head Romaine lettuce, chopped

1 English cucumber, sliced

Directions:

1. Add oyster sauce, Worcestershire sauce, oil, black pepper and salt into a large mixing bowl.
2. Place the turkey breast into the marinade.
3. Refrigerate and marinate for an hour.
4. Grease the air fryer basket with some olive oil.
5. Preheat the air fryer to 380F.
6. Place the chicken breast into the prepared basket and cook for 20 minutes, turning the breast about every 10 minutes with tong to make sure turkey breast are evenly browned.
7. Once the turkey is nice golden brown, transfer it to a cutting board and shred it with the help of two forks to "pull" it apart.

For Assembling:

8. Place the shredded turkey over the toasted bread.
9. Top with a slice of cheese, lettuce and cucumber.
10. Cover with another slice, secure with the toothpick and serve.

Apricot Glazed Turkey Legs

Serving: 4 **Cooking time: 30 minutes**

Nutritional values

Calories 1300 kcal

Fat 61.94 g

Total Carbs 15.87 g

Protein 159.83 g

Ingredients

4 turkey legs, bone-in, skin-on

1/2 cup apricot juice

2 tbsp honey

1 tbsp corn flour

1 tbsp Italian seasoning

1 tsp dried thyme

2 tbsp oil

Salt to taste

For Garnishing:

2 tbsp chives, sliced

Directions:

1. Gather the turkey legs and all the ingredients to a large mixing bowl.
2. Using your clean hands generously rub the spices onto each side of the leg.
3. Preheat the air fryer to 400F.
4. Place the legs into the air fryer basket and cook for 30 minutes, flipping halfway and brushing very lightly with some more oil.
5. Once the legs are golden and sticky, transfer to a serving plate.
6. Garnish with chives and serve hot.

Turkey Meatloaf

Serving: 6　　**Cooking time: 40 minutes**

Nutritional values

Calories 225 kcal

Fat 9.06 g

Total Carbs 13.21 g

Protein 23.73 g

Ingredients

1.5lb. ground turkey

1 small onion, finely chopped

1 cup carrot, shredded

1 cup mushrooms, sliced

1 cup green bell pepper, chopped

2 clove garlic, minced

3 tbsp tomato sauce

1 tbsp Worcestershire sauce

1 tsp cumin

1 tsp black pepper

Salt to taste

For Glaze:

1/4 cup tomato sauce

2 tbsp honey

2 tbsp chili sauce

1 tbsp Dijon mustard

Directions:

1. In a large mixing bowl, combine all the ingredients.
2. Using your hands work the mixture together; mix until all the ingredients are evenly combined.
3. Grease the air fryer basket with non-stick spray or olive oil.
4. Preheat air fryer to 390F.
5. Shape the turkey mixture into a pretty looking meat loaf.
6. Smooth the edges with the back of a spoon.
7. Carefully place the meat loaf in air fryer and cook for 30 minutes.
8. While meatloaf is cooking, mix all the glaze ingredients together in a small mixing bowl.
9. Once the meatloaf is done, brush the glaze all over meatloaf in air fryer.
10. Reduce the temperature to 300F and continue cooking about 10 minutes or until the glaze gets sticky and brown.
11. Remove from the air fryer and let rest at room temperature before slicing and serving.

Cheese Stuffed Turkey Meatballs

Serving: 8　　**Cooking time: 20 minutes**

Nutritional values

Calories 142 kcal

Fat 8.65 g

Total Carbs 3.84 g

Protein 12.61 g

Ingredients

1lb. ground turkey

1 medium onion, finely chopped

2 clove garlic, minced

1 tsp ground ginger

1/4 cup fresh mint leaves, chopped

1/4 cup fresh parsley leaves, chopped

3/4 cup breadcrumbs

1 large egg

1 tsp paprika

1 tsp oregano

2 tbsp oil

Salt to taste

For Filling:

Mozzarella cheese, cut into 20 bite size pieces

Directions:

1. In a large bowl, combine all the ingredients.
2. Shape the mixture into 20 meatballs.
3. Insert 1 mozzarella cube into the center of each meatball; make sure to seal the meat tightly around the cheese.
4. Preheat air fryer to 360F.
5. Cook in the air fryer for 20 minutes.
6. Serve hot.

Turkey Burgers

Serving: 6 **Cooking time: 30 minutes**

Nutritional values

Calories 194 kcal

Fat 9.63 g

Total Carbs 2.67 g

Protein 24.28 g

Ingredients

1.5lb. ground turkey

1 jalapeno, finely chopped

1 cup mushrooms, chopped

1 clove garlic, minced

1 large egg

1/4 cup bread crumbs

1 tbsp teriyaki sauce

Salt & black pepper to tastes

For Filling:

6 Hamburger buns or English muffins

Mayonnaise

Dijon mustard

Lettuce

Tomatoes

6 cheese slices

Directions:

1. In a large bowl, mix together turkey, jalapeno, mushrooms, garlic, egg, bread crumbs, teriyaki sauce, salt and pepper.

2. Divide the meat mixture into 6 even patties.

3. Preheat the air fryer to 360F. Grease the air fryer basket with olive oil.

4. Place the patties in the air fryer and cook for 30 minutes, flipping the patties halfway through.

For Assembling:

5. Spread a spoonful of mustard and mayonnaise onto the bun.

6. Once cooked, immediately place the hot patties onto the prepared bun.

7. Top each Pattie with a slice of cheese, lettuce & tomato.

8. Cover with another bun and serve.

Turkey Sausages

Serving: 10 **Cooking time: 35 minutes**

Nutritional values

Calories 447 kcal

Fat 40.9 g

Total Carbs 0.48 g

Protein 18.07 g

Ingredients

2lb. ground turkey

3/4 cup green onion

1/4 cup parsley, chopped

1 tsp ground sage

1 large egg

Salt to taste

Directions:

1. In a large mixing bowl, crumble the turkey.

2. Add green onion, parsley, egg, ground sage and salt; mix until well combined.

3. Form the mixture into 12 long sausages.

4. Preheat air fryer to 400F.

5. Place the sausages in the air fryer and cook for 35 minutes, turning with spatula halfway through, as needed.

6. Once the sausages temperature reaches 165F, remove from the air fryer.

7. Serve with your favorite dip.

Pork

Buttery Pork Chops

Serving: 4   **Cooking time: 15 minutes**

Nutritional values

Calories 310 kcal

Fat 15.37 g

Total Carbs 1.74 g

Protein 39.56 g

Ingredients

4 bone-in pork chops

3 clove garlic, minced

1 tbsp oregano

1 tsp paprika

1 tsp black pepper

3 tbsp butter

Salt to taste

For Garnishing:

¼ cup green onion, chopped

Directions:

1. Preheat the air fryer to 400F for 8 minutes.

2. In a mixing bowl, combine butter, garlic, oregano, paprika, black pepper, salt.

3. Coat the pork chop with the rub.

4. Place the pork chops into the air fryer basket and cook for 15 minutes, flipping half way through.

5. Garnish with green onion and serve.

BBQ Pulled Pork with Coleslaw

Serving: 6   **Cooking time: 20 minutes**

Nutritional values

Calories 429 kcal

Fat 18.01 g

Total Carbs 21.02 g

Protein 43.23 g

Ingredients

3 lbs. pork shoulder

For Coleslaw:

1 cup mayonnaise

1 cup cabbage, shredded

1/2 cup carrots, shredded

1 tsp sugar

Salt and black pepper to taste

For Rub:

1 cup BBQ sauce

1 tsp garlic powder

1 tbsp chili powder

1 tsp paprika

1/4 tsp cinnamon powder

2 tbsp olive oil

1 tsp black pepper

1 tsp salt

Directions:

For Coleslaw:

1. Mix all the coleslaw ingredients to a small serving bowl and set aside.

For Rub:

2. In a large mixing bowl, combine all the rub ingredients.

3. Add pork and marinate for 3 hours.

4. Preheat the air fryer to 400F.

5. Place the pork in the air fryer basket.

6. Pour the remaining sauce over the top of the pork.

7. Cook for 20 minutes or until internal temperature read 160F.

8. Flip the pork at the halfway cooking point.

9. Once the pork is cooked through, shred it using two forks to "pull" it apart.

10.

Herb Crusted Pork Ribs

Serving: 4   **Cooking time: 25 minutes**

Nutritional values

Calories 838 kcal

Fat 32.41 g

Total Carbs 7.94 g

Protein 119.87 g

Ingredients

5lbs. pork ribs, baby back or spare ribs

1 cup bread crumbs

1 egg

1 tbsp Worcestershire sauce

1 tsp onion powder

1 tsp garlic powder

1 tsp thyme

1 tsp rosemary

1 tsp black pepper

Salt to taste

Directions:

1. Season the pork with salt and black pepper.

2. Place the bread crumbs into a shallow bowl.

3. Add onion powder, garlic powder, thyme, rosemary, black pepper and salt, mix until well combine.

4. Whisk egg and Worcestershire sauce in another bowl.

5. Grab a rib, dunk in the egg and then into the bread crumb mixture.

6. Pat with your hands until they're fully coated.

7. Preheat the air fryer to 400F.

8. Grease the air fryer basket with some oil.

9. Place the ribs into the basket and cook for 25 minutes.

10. Transfer the ribs to a serving plate and serve with your favorite dip.

Balsamic Pork

Serving: 4   **Cooking time: 20 minutes**

Nutritional values

Calories 519 kcal

Fat 11.96 g

Total Carbs 6.34 g

Protein 89.35 g

Ingredients

3lbs. pork tenderloin, cut into four pieces

1/2 cup balsamic vinegar

3 clove garlic, minced

1 tsp oregano

Salt to taste

For Garnishing:

Basil leaves

Directions:

1. Start by preparing a marinade, in a large mixing bowl, combine balsamic vinegar, garlic, oregano and salt.

2. Add the pork pieces and let sit in refrigerator for at least an hour.

3. Preheat the air fryer to 360F.

4. Place the marinated pork into the air fryer basket and cook for 20 minutes.

5. Top with some basil leaves and serve.

Pork Medallions with Sour Cream

Serving: 8   **Cooking time: 10 minutes**

Nutritional values

Calories 212 kcal

Fat 9.38 g

Total Carbs 2.92 g

Protein 27.52 g

Ingredients

2 pork tenderloin, cut into 8 pieces

1/4 cup bread crumbs

1 cup parmesan cheese

2 clove garlic, minced

2 tbsp olive oil

1 tsp black pepper

Salt to taste

For Sour Cream:

1/2 cup sour cream

1 tsp lemon juice

1 tsp black pepper

Directions:

For Sour Cream:

1. Mix all the sour cream ingredients to a bowl and set aside.

For Pork:

2. Slice the pork into 8 pieces; press each piece with the palm of your hand to flatten to 1/4-inch thickness.

3. Rub olive oil and garlic onto each side of the pork.

4. Season the pork with some salt and pepper.

5. In a large shallow dish, combine the bread crumbs and parmesan cheese.

6. Now add pork pieces, 1 slice at a time, to coat evenly.

7. Preheat the air fryer to 400F.

8. Place the pork pieces into the air fryer basket and cook for 10 minutes.

9. Serve with sour cream.

Pork Shoulder Skewers with Pineapple

Serving: 6   **Cooking time: 25 minutes**

Nutritional values

FOR PORK:

Calories 313 kcal

Fat 13.36 g

Total Carbs 17.98 g

Protein 28.96 g

FOR SAUCE:

Calories 25 kcal

Fat 0.08 g

Total Carbs 5.97 g

Protein 0.23 g

Ingredients

2 lbs. pork shoulder, preferably Boston Butt skinless-boneless, cut into 20 pieces

1 tsp garlic powder

1 tsp onion powder

1 cup pineapple juice

1 cup pineapple, chunks

1 tsp oregano

2 tbsp oil

Salt to taste

8 wooden skewers (soaked in cold water for 30 minutes)

For Pineapple Sauce:

1 cup pineapple sauce

1/2 tsp oregano

1 tsp black pepper

1 tsp corn flour

Directions:

1. Whisk pineapple juice, garlic powder, onion powder, oregano, oil and salt in a bowl.

2. Place the pork into the marinade, and let marinate for overnight for a flavorful marination.

3. Preheat the air fryer to 400F.

4. Thread a piece of pork then pineapple onto skewers.

5. Place the skewers into the air fryer basket and cook for 15 minutes.

6. While the pork is cooking prepare the sauce.

7. Place all the sauce ingredients to small pot and bring it to simmer on low heat for about 10 minutes or until it is thicken.

8. Remove from heat.

9. Serve the pork skewers with the sauce.

Pork Steaks with Broccoli

Serving: 4   **Cooking time: 25 minutes**

Nutritional values

Calories 318 kcal

Fat 10.54 g

Total Carbs 11.43 g

Protein 42.61 g

Ingredients

4 boneless pork loin chops, 1/2-inch thick

2 cup broccoli florets

3 clove garlic, minced

1 tsp onion powder

1 tbsp soy sauce

2 tbsp honey

1 tbsp olive oil

Salt to taste

Directions:

1. Combine pork chops, garlic, onion powder, soy sauce, honey, oil and salt to a bowl.

2. Let marinade for 3 hours.

3. Preheat air fryer to 380F.

4. Place the pork in the air fryer and cook for 15 minutes.

5. Once the pork is cooked through, remove from the air fryer.

6. Place the broccoli florets into the air fryer and cook for 5 minutes.

7. Serve the steaks with the broccoli.

Crispy Pork

Serving: 6   **Cooking time: 15 minutes**

Nutritional values

Calories 467 kcal

Fat 19.3 g

Total Carbs 11.55 g

Protein 57.95 g

Ingredients

6 boneless pork loin chops

2 cup bread crumbs

1 cup parmesan cheese, grated

2 large eggs

1 tsp onion powder

1 tsp garlic powder

1 tsp chili powder

1 tsp oregano

1 tsp paprika

Salt to taste

Directions:

1. Preheat the air fryer to 400F and lightly spray the air fryer basket with some oil.

2. In a small mixing bowl, mix onion powder, garlic powder, chili powder, oregano, paprika and salt.

3. Rub the prepared seasoning over the entire pork chops.

4. Combine bread crumbs and cheese in a large shallow bowl.

5. Whisk the eggs in another bowl.

6. Dip the pork into the egg and then into the crumb mixture.

7. Place the prepared chops into the basket.

8. Cook for 15 minutes, turning half way through until evenly browned.

9.

Pork Dumplings

Serving: 10   **Cooking time: 12 minutes**

Nutritional values

Calories 262 kcal

Fat 10.34 g

Total Carbs 28.44 g

Protein 12.42 g

Ingredients

1lb. Ground pork

15 dumpling wrappers or wonton wrappers

1/4 cup green onion

2 clove garlic, minced

1 tbsp Worcestershire sauce

1 tsp thyme

Salt to taste

Directions:

1. Stir together ground pork, green onion, garlic, Worcestershire sauce, thyme and salt in a medium bowl.

2. Place a dumpling wrapper on a lightly floured work surface.

3. Add a spoonful of filling in the center of each wrapper.

4. Using your index fingers, moisten the outer edges of the wrapper with water.

5. Press to seal tightly in the center.

6. Preheat the air fryer to 400F and lightly coat the air fryer basket with some oil.

7. Place the dumplings in the air fryer and cook for 12 minutes.

8. Serve the dumplings with your favorite dip.

Pork Quesadillas

Serving: 4   **Cooking time: 25 minutes**

Nutritional values

Calories 201 kcal

Fat 2.89 g

Total Carbs 30.09 g

Protein 13.38 g

Ingredients

1lb. Ground pork

4 flour tortillas, 10 inches

1 medium onion, chopped

1 cup red bell pepper, sliced

1 cup mushrooms, sliced

1 cup mozzarella cheese

1 tbsp oyster sauce

1 tbsp ginger

1 tsp chili sauce

Salt to taste

For Serving:

1 cup salsa

Directions:

1. Combine ground pork, oyster, ginger, chili sauce and salt to a bowl; mix until well combined.

2. Lay out the tortillas and divide the ground pork between each tortilla.

3. Add onion, bell pepper and mushrooms.

4. Sprinkle mozzarella cheese on top and sandwich with second tortilla; fold in half.

5. Preheat the air fryer to 400F.

6. Light grease the air fryer basket.

7. Place the tortillas in the basket and cook for 25 minutes, flipping halfway and brushing very lightly with more oil, until both sides are golden brown and cheese is melted.

8. Serve with salsa.

BBQ Pork Sandwich

Serving: 6 **Cooking time: 20 minutes**

Nutritional values

Calories 436 kcal

Fat 17.34 g

Total Carbs 8.78 g

Protein 57.48 g

Ingredients

4lbs. pork shoulder, skinless

2 tbsp onion powder

2 tbsp garlic powder

1 tbsp dried oregano

1 tsp thyme

2 tbsp sugar

Salt to taste

For Serving:

6 hamburger buns

1 cup coleslaw

1 cup BBQ sauce

1/4 cup Dijon mustard

Directions:

1. Start by preparing a rub; combine all the ingredients to a medium bowl.
2. Rub all over the pork.
3. Cover and let marinate for 4 hours.
4. Preheat the air fryer to 360F.
5. Place the pork into the air fryer basket and cook for 20 minutes or until internal temperature of pork reaches 160F.
6. Remove from the air fryer and let cool at room temperature.
7. Slice the pork.

Assembling:

8. Divide the sliced pork on top of each bun, top with coleslaw, BBQ sauce and Dijon mustard.
9. Add some lettuce leaves and affix the top half of the bun.
10. Slice and serve.

Crispy Coconut Pork Belly

Serving: 4 **Cooking time: 25 minutes**

Nutritional values

Calories 1245 kcal

Fat 127.01 g

Total Carbs 2.89 g

Protein 21.6 g

Ingredients

2lbs. Pork belly, cubed

1/2 cup coconut, shredded

1 tbsp Worcestershire sauce

1 tsp oregano

1 tsp black pepper

1 tbsp coconut oil

Salt to taste

Directions:

1. Add pork belly, Worcestershire sauce, oregano, black pepper, coconut oil and salt to a bowl, mix well.
2. Place the cubes into the shredded coconut and toss, until evenly coated.
3. Preheat the air fryer to 360F.
4. Place the pork in the air fryer and cook for 25 minutes until browned.
5. Serve with your favorite dip.

Lemon Pork Ribs

Serving: 8 **Cooking time: 20 minutes**

Nutritional values

Calories 259 kcal

Fat 11.32 g

Total Carbs 1.59 g

Protein 35.46 g

Ingredients

3 lbs. baby back pork ribs

3 cloves garlic, minced

3 tbsp thyme

3 tbsp lemon juice

1 tsp lemon zest

1 tsp brown sugar

1 tbsp olive oil

Salt to taste

For Garnishing:

1/2 cup fresh parsley, chopped

Directions:

1. Combine garlic, thyme, lemon juice, lemon zest, brown sugar and salt.

2. Smear the paste on each rib.

3. Preheat the air fryer at 360F and grease the basket with oil.

4. Cook ribs for about 20 minutes until golden brown.

5. Garnish with fresh parsley and serve.

Honey Mustard Pork Chops

Serving: 4 **Cooking time: 20 minutes**

Nutritional values

Calories 309 kcal

Fat 6.62 g

Total Carbs 19.03 g

Protein 42.02 g

Ingredients

4 boneless pork loin chops

3 clove garlic, minced

1/4 cup honey

2 tbsp Dijon mustard

1 tsp black pepper

Salt to taste

For Sauce:

1/2 cup tomato sauce

1 tsp Worcestershire sauce

1/2 tsp honey

1 tsp black pepper

Directions:

For Sauce:

1. Mix all the sauce ingredients to a serving bowl & set aside.

For Pork Chops:

2. In a mixing bowl, mix garlic, honey, mustard, black pepper and salt, whisk until well combined.

3. Place the pork in a large zip-loc bag and pour in the prepared mixture.

4. Squish around until completely covered with the mixture. Marinate for 4 hours.

5. Preheat the air fryer to 360F and grease the basket with some oil.

6. Place the marinated pork chops into the air fryer basket and cook for 15 minutes.

7. Turn the chops after 5-7 minutes.

is browned and crisp.

9. Remove from the air fryer and serve with the sauce.

Beef

Teriyaki Beef Steak with Broccoli

Serving: 4   **Cooking time: 20 minutes**

Nutritional values

Calories 907 kcal

Fat 71.81 g

Total Carbs 3.19 g

Protein 62.69 g

Ingredients

3 large beef ribeye or filet mignon steaks

2 cups broccoli florets

3 clove garlic, minced

2 tbsp teriyaki sauce

1 tbsp Worcestershire sauce

1 tsp oregano

Salt to taste

Directions:

1. In a small mixing bowl, combine garlic, teriyaki sauce, Worcestershire sauce, oregano and salt.

2. Pour the marinade over the steak, turn upside down to coat well.

3. Cover and refrigerate for at least 6 hours.

4. Preheat the air fryer to 400F and grease the basket with some oil.

5. Place the steaks in the air fryer and cook for 20 minutes, flip halfway through after 10 minutes for medium rare.

6. Remove the steak from the air fryer and place the broccoli florets in the basket.

7. Cook for 5 minutes.

8. Serve the steak with broccoli.

Beef Chipotle

Serving: 6   **Cooking time: 30 minutes**

Nutritional values

Calories 347 kcal

Fat 15.41 g

Total Carbs 4.52 g

Protein 49.01 g

Ingredients

3lbs. beef chuck steak

2 clove garlic, minced

5 red chili, soaked in vinegar for 2 hours

1/4 cup tomato puree

3 tbsp lemon juice

1 tbsp vinegar

1 tbsp Worcestershire sauce

1 tsp cumin

Salt to taste

For Garnishing:

1/4 cup parsley, chopped

Some lime, sliced

Directions:

1. In a blender add garlic, chili, tomato puree, lemon juice, vinegar, Worcestershire sauce, cumin and salt; blend until well combined.

2. Place the steaks into a shallow dish and pour the marinade on top. Marinate for 4 hours.

3. Preheat the air fryer to 360F.

4. Place the marinated beef into the air fryer basket and cook for 20 minutes.

5. Once the beef is done, remove from the air fryer and let cool at room temperature.

6. Shred the meat with the help of two forks and return it back to the air fryer.

7.

Lemon Herb Beef Roast

Serving: 6 **Cooking time: 50 minutes**

Nutritional values

Calories 376 kcal

Fat 16.98 g

Total Carbs 2.96 g

Protein 53.71 g

Ingredients

3 lbs. beef sirloin roast, boneless

2 cups beef broth

1/4 cup butter

1 tbsp onion powder

2 tsp garlic powder

3 tbsp lemon juice

1 tbsp thyme

1 tbsp basil

1 tbsp oregano

1 tbsp rosemary

1 tsp dried dill

1 tsp black pepper

Salt to taste

Directions:

1. Place the beef in a shallow dish, allowing to come at room temperature.

2. Make a rub by combining lemon juice, onion powder, garlic powder, thyme, basil, oregano, rosemary, dill, black pepper and salt.

3. Rub the mixture all over the beef until evenly coated.

4. Pour the broth, cover and let marinate for at least 6 hours.

5. Grease the air fryer basket with butter and preheat at 400F for 10 minutes.

6. Place the marinated beef into the basket and cook for 30 minutes, flip the roast and continue cooking for another 20 minutes until fall-apart tender.

7. Chop into quarters and serve.

Skirt Steak Fajitas Wraps

Serving: 8 **Cooking time: 25 minutes**

Nutritional values

Calories 231 kcal

Fat 13.74 g

Total Carbs 3.41 g

Protein 23.64 g

Ingredients

2 lbs. trimmed skirt steak, cut into 6 inch crosswise pieces

For Marinade:

2 clove garlic, minced

2 tbsp Worcestershire sauce

1 tbsp taco seasoning

2 tsp ground cumin seeds

1 tbsp chili powder

4 tbsps olive oil

1 tbsp brown sugar

1 tsp ground black pepper

Salt to taste

For Guacamole:

2 large avocados

1/2 small onion, chopped

1/2 cup tomatoes, chopped

1 garlic, minced

1 tbsp lime juice

3 tbsp cilantro, chopped

For Fajitas:

1 cup mozzarella cheese, shredded

¼ cup sour cream

1 large red bell pepper, sliced

1 large yellow bell pepper, sliced

1 large green bell pepper, sliced

1 white onion, sliced

8 tortillas

Directions:

For Guacamole:

1. In a medium mixing bowl, mash avocado, garlic and lime juice.

2. Add in chopped onion, tomatoes and cilantro; mix until well combined.

For Fajitas:

3. Mix all the marinade ingredients to a small mixing bowl.

4. Place the beef in a Ziploc bag and pour the marinade.

5. Marinate for 2 hours.

6. Preheat the air fryer to 360F and grease basket with some oil.

7. Add the marinated beef and sliced peppers to the air fryer and cook at 400F for 20 minutes.

8. Once the beef is cooked through, transfer into a large serving bowl.

9. Spoon about 3 tbsp of the mixture down the center of each tortilla.

10. Add sliced onion and a tbspful of guacamole.

11. Top with some shredded cheese and sour cream; roll up tightly.

12. Place the rolled tortillas, seam side down in the greased air fryer basket and cook for 5 minutes.

13. Serve the wrap warm.

Beef Stuffed Capsicum

Serving: 6   **Cooking time: 15 minutes**

Nutritional values

Calories 338 kcal

Fat 25.22 g

Total Carbs 9.98 g

Protein 18.35 g

Ingredients

1lb. lean ground beef

6 Large Bell Peppers

1 cup mozzarella cheese, shredded

1/2 cup onion, chopped

1 tbsp hot sauce

1 tbsp soy sauce

1 tsp garlic, crushed

1 tbsp olive oil

1 tsp black pepper

1 tsp salt

For Garnishing:

Parsley, chopped

Lemon slices

Directions:

1. Cut the capsicums in half and discard the ribs and seeds.

2. Combine ground beef, onion, hot sauce, soy sauce, garlic, oil, black pepper and salt in a large mixing bowl.

3. Lightly grease the air fryer basket and preheat at 360F.

4. Stuff each pepper with the meat mixture and sprinkle with mozzarella cheese.

5. Carefully place the peppers into the air fryer basket and cook for 15 minutes or until tender.

6. Garnish with parsley and sliced lemon.

Spaghetti Meatballs on Stick

Serving: 10   **Cooking time: 15 minutes**

Nutritional values

Calories 179 kcal

Fat 15.52 g

Total Carbs 1.93 g

Protein 7.45 g

Ingredients

1lb. lean ground beef

1 small onion, chopped

1 tsp garlic, crushed

1 bread slice, crumbled

1/4 cup basil, chopped

1 large egg

1 tbsp olive oil

Salt and pepper to taste

For Serving:

1 package of spaghetti

1 cup pizza sauce

15 wooden skewers

Directions:

1. In a large mixing bowl, combine beef, onion, garlic, bread slice, basil, egg, salt and pepper. Mix until well combined.

2. Using your hands or a small scoop make 1-inch sized meatballs.

3. Preheat the air fryer to 400F and grease the air fryer basket with oil.

4. Place the meatballs into the air fryer basket and cook for 15 minutes.

5. While the meatballs are cooking, cook spaghetti according to the package instructions.

6. Once the meatballs are done, remove from the fryer.

7. Twirl 8-10 spaghetti strands around skewer and insert into meatball.

8. Add a spoonful of pizza sauce on top and serve.

Salted Beef with Caramelized Onions

Serving: 6 **Cooking time: 40 minutes**

Nutritional values

Calories 310 kcal

Fat 17.5 g

Total Carbs 4.35 g

Protein 31.7 g

Ingredients

2lbs. beef top sirloin steak

1 tbsp Worcestershire sauce

Salt and pepper to taste

For Caramelized Onions:

1 large onion, thinly sliced into rings

1 tsp butter

1 tsp brown sugar

Directions:

For Caramelized Onion:

1. Mix all the ingredients to a large mixing bowl and set aside.

For Beef:

2. In a large mixing bowl, mix Worcestershire sauce, salt and pepper.

3. Add the beef and marinate for 2 hours.

4. Preheat the air fryer to 400F.

5. Place the marinated beef in the air fryer basket and cook for 20 minutes.

6. Once the time is up, place the onion over the top of the beef and set timer for another 20 minutes.

7. Serve the beef hot.

Sticky BBQ Honey Strips

Serving: 4 **Cooking time: 15 minutes**

Nutritional values

Calories 543 kcal

Fat 22.91 g

Total Carbs 47.46 g

Protein 36.01 g

Ingredients

1.5lbs. beef top sirloin steak, cut into ¼ inch thick strips

1 cup BBQ sauce

1/4 cup honey

1 tsp Dijon mustard

1 tsp hot sauce

1 tsp oregano

1 tsp paprika

1 tbsp oil

Salt to taste

For Garnishing:

1/4 cup parsley, chopped

Directions:

1. In a medium bowl, whisk BBQ sauce, honey, mustard, hot sauce, oregano, paprika and salt.

2. Add beef and marinate for 30 minutes.

3. Preheat the air fryer to 400F and grease the basket with oil.

4. Add beef to the air fryer and cook for 15 minutes.

5. Garnish the beef with chopped parsley and serve.

Beef with Mix Vegetables

Serving: 6   **Cooking time: 20 minutes**

Nutritional values

Calories 604 kcal

Fat 38.72 g

Total Carbs 30.83 g

Protein 35.79 g

Ingredients

2lbs. beef tenderloin, cut into cubes

1 cup carrots, sliced

1 cup cabbage, sliced

1 cup green bell pepper, sliced

1 cup corn

1 tbsp butter

1 tbsp soy sauce

1 tbsp Worcestershire sauce

1 tbsp cream

1 tsp oregano

1/2 tsp red chili flakes

1 tsp black pepper

Salt to taste

For Serving:

Boiled rice

Directions:

1. Mix all the vegetables to a bowl and season with some salt and pepper.

2. In a medium bowl, mix butter, soy sauce, Worcestershire sauce, cream, oregano, chili flakes and salt.

3. Add in the cubed beef and let marinate for 20 minutes.

4. Preheat the air fryer to 360F.

5. Place the marinated beef into the air fryer and cook for 10 minutes.

6. Once the beef is cooked through remove from the fryer and set aside.

7. Place all the vegetables into the same basket and cook for 5 minutes.

8. Add the beef back to the vegetables and cook for additional 5 minutes.

9. Serve the beef and vegetables with boiled rice.

Crispy Mongolian Beef

Serving: 6   **Cooking time: 15 minutes**

Nutritional values

Calories 281 kcal

Fat 14.95 g

Total Carbs 5 g

Protein 32.87 g

Ingredients

2lbs. beef tenderloin or beef chuck, cut into strips

3 tbsp corn flour

1/4 cup sesame seeds (optional)

1 tbsp soy sauce

1 tbsp vinegar

1 tbsp oyster sauce

1 tsp brown sugar

1 tsp red chili flakes

1 tbsp oil

For Garnishing:

1/4 cup green onion, chopped

Directions:

1. Start off by mixing the beef with soy sauce, vinegar, oyster sauce, brown sugar and chili flakes in a bowl.

2. Sprinkle corn flour and sesame seeds; mix until the strips are coated evenly.

3. Preheat the air fryer to 400F.

4. Grease the air fryer basket with oil and cook for about 15 minutes, flipping the strips halfway through.

5. Garnish with green onion and serve.

Thai Beef Salad

Serving: 4 **Cooking time: 12 minutes**

Nutritional values

Calories 528 kcal

Fat 32.33 g

Total Carbs 7.21 g

Protein 50.68 g

Ingredients

1.5lb. beef sirloin steaks, slice into thin strips

3 clove garlic, minced

1 tsp ginger, grated

1 tbsp fish sauce

2 tsps sesame oil

For Salad:

1 medium head lettuce, chopped

2 carrots, sliced

1 cup cherry tomatoes, sliced in half

1 large cucumber, sliced

1 jalapeno pepper, minced

1 cup bell pepper, thinly sliced

2 tbsp lemon juice

1/4 cup peanuts

Directions:

1. In a large mixing bowl, combine, garlic, ginger, fish sauce and sesame oil.

2. Add beef strips and marinate for 2 hours.

3. Preheat the air fryer to 400F.

4. Place the marinated beef in the air fryer and cook for 12 minutes.

5. Once the beef is done, let cool at room temperature.

6. Meanwhile in a large serving bowl, combine all the vegetables.

7. Add beef and lemon juice, toss well.

8. Top with peanuts and serve.

Chinese Beef and Broccoli

Serving: 4 **Cooking time: 15 minutes**

Nutritional values

Calories 275 kcal

Fat 16.38 g

Total Carbs 5.04 g

Protein 26.18 g

Ingredients

1lbs. beef flank or sirloin steak, cut into thin pieces

1/2lb. broccoli, cut into bite-size florets

3 clove garlic, minced

1 tsp ginger, grated

2 tbsp soy sauce

2 tbsp balsamic vinegar

1 tsp corn flour

1 tbsp oil

1 tsp black pepper

Salt to taste

For Garnishing:

1/4 cup cilantro, chopped

Directions:

1. Mix all the ingredients together in a bowl, toss until well mixed.

2. Preheat the air fryer to 400F.

3. Add the beef and broccoli in the air fryer and cook for 15 minutes.

4. Garnish with chopped cilantro and serve.

Beef Kabobs

Serving: 10 **Cooking time: 15 minutes**

Nutritional values

Calories 224 kcal

Fat 14.79 g

Total Carbs 2.63 g

Protein 19.48 g

Ingredients

2lbs. beef sirloin cut into 1 inch-pieces

1/4 cup butter

1 cup onion, cut into 1-inch pieces

1 large green bell pepper, cut into 1-inch pieces

1 cup mushrooms

1 cup zucchini, sliced into discs

3 clove garlic

Salt and pepper to taste

12 wooden skewers

For Serving:

1/4 cup sour cream

Directions:

1. Preheat the air fryer to 400F.
2. Mix garlic, salt and pepper to butter.
3. Thread a piece of beef, onion, bell pepper, mushrooms and zucchini onto the skewers.
4. Follow the same sequence until the skewer is filled till top.
5. Brush each skewer with the butter and garlic mixture.
6. Place the skewers in the air fryer and cook for 15 minutes, flipping halfway and brushing very lightly with more butter (if needed).
7. Serve the kabobs with sour cream.

Beef & Mushroom Meatloaf

Serving: 6 **Cooking time: 25 minutes**

Nutritional values

Calories 154 kcal

Fat 6.37 g

Total Carbs 5.03 g

Protein 19.19 g

Ingredients

1lb. ground beef

1 cup mushrooms, sliced

1/2 cup parmesan cheese

1/2 cup pizza sauce

3 clove garlic, minced

2 tbsp Worcestershire sauce

1 tbsp lemon juice

Salt and pepper to taste

For Garnishing:

1/4 cup parsley, chopped

Directions:

1. Preheat air fryer to 400F.
2. Grease a loaf tin with some butter.
3. Combine ground beef and mushrooms in a bowl.
4. Add in the remaining ingredients, mix until well combined.
5. Add the meat mixture into the prepared pan.
6. Place the meatloaf tin in the air fryer and cook for 25 minutes.
7. Garnish with chopped parsley, slice and serve.

Lamb

Roasted Lamb Leg

Serving: 8   **Cooking time: 30 minutes**

Nutritional values

Calories 338 kcal

Fat 11.42 g

Total Carbs 21.4 g

Protein 38.42 g

Ingredients

3-4 lbs. lamb leg

5-6 potatoes cut into chunks

1 cup peas

3 clove garlic, minced

2 tsp oregano

2 tsp rosemary

2 tsp black pepper

2 tbsp olive oil

Salt to taste

For Garnishing:

3-4 lemon slices

1/4 cup parsley, chopped

Directions:

1. Preheat air fryer to 400F.

2. With the help of sharp knife mark slits in the lamb.

3. Rub the lamb leg with garlic, oregano, rosemary, black pepper, oil and salt.

4. Line the air fryer basket with foil.

5. Place the lamb, potatoes and peas in the basket and cook for 30 minutes.

6. Garnish with parsley and lemon slices.

Lemon Herb Lamb Chops

Serving: 4   **Cooking time: 10 minutes**

Nutritional values

Calories 124 kcal

Fat 5.84 g

Total Carbs 1.31 g

Protein 16.88 g

Ingredients

8 lamb chops

1/4 cup lemon juice

1 tsp rosemary

1 tsp oregano

1 tsp thyme

Salt to taste

Directions:

1. Preheat air fryer to 400F.

2. Season the chops with rosemary, oregano, thyme and salt.

3. Pour in the lemon juice and let marinate for 20 minutes.

4. Place the marinated chops in the air fryer and roast for 10 minutes until nicely brown. Serve warm.

Lamb Steak with Sweet Potatoes

Serving: 6   **Cooking time: 12 minutes**

Nutritional values

Calories 343 kcal

Fat 11.5 g

Total Carbs 10.58 g

Protein 49.19 g

Ingredients

3lbs. lamb leg steaks- bone-in

2 large sweet potato, cubed

1/4 cup red/white wine vinegar

2 tbsp soy sauce

1 tbsp hoisin sauce

1 tbsp mustard

1 tsp olive oil

Salt and pepper to taste

For Sauce:

1 cup tomato sauce

1 tbsp soy sauce

1 tbsp Worcestershire sauce

1 tsp brown sugar

Directions:

For Sauce:

1. Mix all the ingredients to a bowl and microwave for 5 minutes until thick; set aside.

For Lamb:

2. Rub the lamb steaks with little olive oil.

3. Mix vinegar, soy sauce, hoisin sauce, mustard paste, salt and pepper to a mixing bowl.

4. Coat the steaks with the prepared mixture; marinate for 30 minutes.

5. Preheat the air fryer to 360F.

6. Grease the air fryer basket with some oil.

7. Place the steaks and sweet potatoes in the basket and cook for 12 minutes, flip after 6 minutes to evenly brown.

8. Once browned, transfer the steaks and potatoes to a serving dish.

9. Drizzle with sauce and serve.

Thai Lamb Stir Fry

Serving: 8   **Cooking time: 15 minutes**

Nutritional values

Calories 471 kcal

Fat 40.04 g

Total Carbs 6.5 g

Protein 21.63 g

Ingredients

2lbs. lamb fillet or back strap, cut into strips

1 cup red bell pepper, cut into strips

1 cup mushrooms, sliced

1 cup cashews

1/4 cup coconut milk

1 tbsp fish sauce

1 tbsp curry paste

1 tsp brown sugar

1 tbsp peanut oil

For Garnishing:

1/4 cup cilantro, chopped

Directions:

1. Combine lamb strips, coconut milk, fish sauce, curry paste, brown sugar and oil to a mixing bowl; cover and place in the refrigerator for 2 hours.

2. Preheat the air fryer to 400F.

3. Place the marinated lamb, veggies and cashews into the basket.

4. Cook for 15 minutes.

5. Garnish with cilantro and serve.

Classic Lamb Shanks

Serving: 4　　**Cooking time: 30 minutes**

Nutritional values

Calories 427 kcal

Fat 26.6 g

Total Carbs 14.35 g

Protein 32.06 g

Ingredients

4 medium lamb shanks

2 cup beef or chicken broth

1/4 cup tomato sauce

3 clove garlic, minced

1 tsp ginger, grated

1 tbsp soy sauce

1 tbsp Worcestershire sauce

2 tbsp olive oil

Salt and pepper to taste

For Serving:

2 lime, sliced

Directions:

1. Place the lamb shanks in a shallow dish.
2. Blend all the ingredients in a blender and pour over the lamb.
3. Using your hands, generously rub the marinade onto each side of the lamb.
4. Cover and refrigerate for 2 hours.
5. Preheat the air fryer to 400F.
6. Place the lamb shanks into the air fryer basket and cook for 20 minutes.
7. Turn the lamb once while roasting.
8. Transfer the remaining marinade to a pot and let simmer on low heat for about 10 minutes.
9. Once the lamb shanks are cooked through, remove from the fryer and immediately pour the sauce over the shanks. Serve with sliced lime.

Basil Lamb Cutlets

Serving: 6　　**Cooking time: 15 minutes**

Nutritional values

Calories 326 kcal

Fat 27.61 g

Total Carbs 2.23 g

Protein 15.83 g

Ingredients

6 lamb cutlets

1/4 cup balsamic vinegar

1 cup basil leaves, chopped

1/2 cup parsley, chopped

1 tbsp olive oil

Salt to taste

For Garnishing:

A handful of fresh basil leaves

Directions:

1. In a blender blend all the ingredients together until smooth.
2. Transfer the marinade to a large mixing bowl.
3. Add the cutlets and let sit in refrigerator for at least one hour.
4. Preheat the air fryer to 360F.
5. Place the cutlets in the air fryer and cook for 15 minutes, turning over once halfway through.
6. Arrange basil leaves in a large serving dish.
7. Place the cutlets over the basil leaves and serve.

Lamb Pie

Serving: 4   **Cooking time: 30 minutes**

Nutritional values

Calories 629 kcal   Total Carbs 36.56 g

Fat 38.99 g   Protein 33.12 g

Ingredients

1lb. ground lamb

1 pie-crust pastry

1 cup pizza sauce

1 cup cheddar cheese

1/4 cup onion, chopped

1/4 cup green onion, chopped

1 tsp oregano

1 tsp black pepper

Salt to taste

Directions:

1. Preheat air fryer to 360F and grease a pie dish with some butter.

2. In a large mixing bowl, combine lamb, onion, green onion, oregano, black pepper and salt. Mix until well combined.

3. Meanwhile on a lightly floured surface, roll the dough into two large rounds.

4. Transfer the dough to the prepared pie dish and gently press with the palm of your hands.

5. Add the marinated lamb and top with a layer of pizza sauce and cheese.

6. Cover it with the remaining rolled dough.

7. With the help of a knife mark 4 slits to let steam escape.

8. Place the pie in the air fryer and cook for 30 minutes until nice golden brown.

Mediterranean Lamb Burgers

Serving: 6   **Cooking time: 12 minutes**

Nutritional values

Calories 170 kcal   Total Carbs 4.54 g

Fat 9.67 g   Protein 16.2 g

Ingredients

1lb. ground lamb

2 bread slices, crumbled

1 tsp garlic powder

1 tsp onion powder

1/4 cup mint leaves, chopped

1 tsp paprika

1 tsp hot sauce

Salt to taste

For Topping:

6 pita pockets

1/2 cup sour cream

1 head Romaine lettuce, chopped

1 large tomato, sliced

Cucumber, sliced

Black olives, pitted and sliced

Directions:

1. Combine ground lamb and all the ingredients to a mixing bowl and knead well.

2. Form the mixture into 6 large patties.

3. Preheat air fryer to 360F and grease the basket with some oil.

4. Place the Patties, 3 at a time in the fryer and cook for 12 minutes, 6 minutes on each side or until well done.

For Assembling:

5. Assemble each pita pockets with a Pattie and some lettuce.

6. Top with sliced tomatoes, cucumber and olives.

7. Serve with a dollop of sour cream and serve.

Sweet and Sour Lamb Ribs

Serving: 4 **Cooking time: 20 minutes**

Nutritional values

Calories 477 kcal

Fat 21.45 g

Total Carbs 22.86 g

Protein 45.93 g

Ingredients

2lbs. lamb ribs

8 sprigs fresh rosemary,

3 clove garlic, minced

2 tsp ginger, grated

1/4 cup honey

4 tbsp balsamic vinegar

1 tsp chili flakes

Salt to taste

Directions:

1. Mix garlic, ginger, honey, vinegar, chili flakes and salt to a mixing bowl.

2. Brush the marinade all over the ribs.

3. Place ribs and rosemary in the air fryer and cook for 20 minutes, flip and brown the other side for 10 minutes, brushing with more marinade.

4. Once the ribs are nice golden brown, remove from the fryer and serve hot.

Spicy Lamb Meatballs with Mango Salsa

Serving: 12 **Cooking time: 15 minutes**

Nutritional values

FOR MEATBALLS:

Calories 97 kcal

Fat 5.02 g

Total Carbs 4.47 g

Protein 8.5 g

FOR SALSA:

Calories 48 kcal

Fat 0.61 g

Total Carbs 11.08 g

Protein 0.95 g

Ingredients

1lb. ground lamb

1 medium onion, finely chopped

1/2 cup tomatoes, chopped

1/2 cup zucchini, chopped

1 clove garlic, minced

1 tsp ginger, grated

2 bread slices, crumbled

1/2 cup marinara sauce

1 tbsp Italian seasoning

2 tsp green chilies, chopped

Salt to taste

For Mango Salsa:

1 cup mango, chopped

1/4 cup tomato chopped

1/4 cup cucumber chopped

1 tsp lemon juice

2 tbsps pomegranate seeds

Directions:

For Mango Salsa:

1. Mix all the salsa ingredients to a small serving bowl and set aside.

For Meatballs:

2. Mix all the ingredients to a mixing bowl.

3. Using your hands work the mixture together; mix until all the ingredients are evenly combined.

4. Shape the mixture into 15 meatballs and place onto a baking sheet; refrigerate for 2 hours.

5.

for 15 minutes until golden brown.

Walnut-Stuffed Lamb

Serving: 8   **Cooking time: 30 minutes**

Nutritional values

Calories 433 kcal

Fat 36.95 g

Total Carbs 2.69 g

Protein 22.28 g

Ingredients

2lbs. lamb breasts, boneless

1 tsp olive oil

Salt

For Stuffing:

1 cup cream cheese

1 cup spinach, chopped

1/2 cup walnuts, chopped

1/3 cup parsley, coarsely chopped

3 tbsps fresh lemon juice

1 tsp oregano

Salt and pepper to taste

Directions:

1. Start off by preparing the stuffing. Mix all the stuffing ingredients to a bowl and set aside.

2. Flatten lamb to 1/4-inch thickness.

3. Rub the breast with oil and salt.

4. Spread the stuffing mixture evenly over both lamb breast.

5. Working with the short end, roll up the breast tightly, tying each roll with kitchen twine at even intervals.

6. Preheat the air fryer to 400F.

7. Carefully place the roll in the air fryer and cook for 30 minutes, turning occasionally until browned on all sides.

8. Once the rolls are cooked, remove from the fryer.

9. Slice and serve.

Plum Roast Lamb

Serving: 6   **Cooking time: 30 minutes**

Nutritional values

Calories 332 kcal

Fat 21.98 g

Total Carbs 5.42 g

Protein 28.48 g

Ingredients

2lbs. lamb, shoulder, leg or shank

1 cup plum sauce or plums soaked in water

1 tbsp honey or molasses

1 tsp Worcestershire sauce

1 tbsp soy sauce

1 tsp black pepper

Salt to taste

Garnishing:

1/2 cup parsley, chopped

Directions:

1. Mix all ingredients together in a small bowl.

2. Pour the marinade over the lamb, cover and refrigerate for 3 hours.

3. Preheat the air fryer to 400F and cook the lamb for 30 minutes or until falling off the bone.

4. Remove from the air fryer, garnish with parsley and serve.

Turkish Kebabs with Tahini Sauce

Serving: 8　　**Cooking time: 8 minutes**

Nutritional values

FOR KEBABS:

Calories 414 kcal
Fat 35.6 g
Total Carbs 5.99 g
Protein 18.28 g

FOR TAHINI SAUCE:

Calories 75 kcal
Fat 7.44 g
Total Carbs 1.26 g
Protein 1.95 g

Ingredients

2 lbs. lamb, cut into 1-inch cubes
1/4 cup butter
1 cup onion, cubed
1 cup potatoes, cubed
1 tsp onion powder
1 tsp garlic powder
2 tbsp oregano
1 tsp thyme
1 tsp rosemary
1 tsp paprika
1 tsp chili powder
3-5 strands of saffron, soaked in 1/4 cup of milk

8 wooden skewers

For Tahini Sauce:

1/2 cup sesame seeds
1 clove garlic
1/4 cup warm water
1 tbsp olive oil
1/4 tsp paprika
Salt to taste

For Serving:

8 pita bread
1 lemon wedges
Salt to taste

Directions:

For Tahini:

1. Add sesame seeds, garlic, water and salt to a blender and blend until thick and creamy consistency. Transfer the sauce to a serving bowl, drizzle some olive oil and sprinkle some paprika on top.

For Kebabs:

2. In a large mixing bowl, combine lamb and all the spices together; toss until evenly coated.

3. Alternately thread a lamb cube, a piece of onion and potato onto skewers, repeat until finished will all.

4. Preheat the air fryer to 400F.

5. Brush the skewers with butter and cook for 6 to 8 minutes, turning occasionally until the lamb and veggies are cooked through.

6. Garnish with lemon wedges and serve with tahini sauce and pita bread.

Crispy Cheesy Lamb Chops

Serving: 6　　**Cooking time: 15 minutes**

Nutritional values

Calories 268 kcal　　Total Carbs 6.44 g

Fat 13.29 g　　Protein 30.77 g

Ingredients

6 lamb chops, bone-in

1 cup bread crumbs

1 cup parmesan cheese

1 tsp oregano

1 large egg

1 tbsp olive oil

Salt and pepper to taste

Directions:

1. Season the chops with salt and pepper.

2. In a shallow dish, combine bread crumbs, cheese and oregano.

3. In another mixing bowl, whisk egg and oil until frothy.

4. Dip each chop in the egg and then into the breadcrumb mixture. Using your hands pat the crumb mixture on chops until evenly coated.

5. Preheat the air fryer to 360F and cook chops for 15 minutes, turn the chops once while cooking.

6. Serve with your favorite sauce.

Vegetarian

Blooming Onion with Spicy Dip

Serving: 12 **Cooking time: 15 minutes**

Nutritional values

Calories 45 kcal

Fat 2.01 g

Total Carbs 5.06 g

Protein 2.09 g

Ingredients

1 large onion, preferably
Vidalia onion
1 cup bread crumbs
1 tsp onion powder
1 tsp garlic powder
2 tbsps paprika
1/2 tsp dried thyme
1/2 tsp dried oregano
For Batter:
1/2 cup milk
2 large eggs

2 tbsp corn flour
1/2 tbsp oil
1 tsp salt
For Spicy Dip:
1 cup mayonnaise
2 tbsp tomato sauce
1 tsp onion powder
1 tsp paprika
1/2 tsp sugar
Pinch of chili flakes

Directions:

For Dip:
1. Mix all the ingredients together and set aside.

For Onion:
2. Wash the onion thoroughly and trim the one end off.
3. Set it on flat surface and start cutting downwards to form into a blossom shape.
4. Soak the onion in ice water for at least an hour or overnight to separate the petals.
5. In a mixing bowl, combine bread crumbs, onion powder, garlic powder, paprika, thyme, oregano and salt.
6. In another separate bowl, whisk together eggs, milk and corn flour together.
7. Carefully place the onion into the egg batter. Spoon on top if necessary.
8. Remove from the batter, letting excess drip off.
9. Immediately transfer the onion into the bread crumb mixture, using your hands pat the bread crumbs onto each side of the onion until they are fully covered.
10. Add oil to the bottom of the air fryer and preheat to 400F.
11. Place the onion into the air fryer basket and cook for 15 minutes or until golden and crispy.
12. Once done, carefully remove from the air fryer & serve with the dip.

Cheesy Jalapenos

Serving: 6 **Cooking time: 10 minutes**

Nutritional values

Calories 221 kcal

Fat 7.18 g

Total Carbs 28.73 g

Protein 10.17 g

Ingredients

6 large jalapeño peppers

1 cup cheddar cheese, shredded

1 cup all-purpose flour

2 cup bread crumbs

2 eggs

1 tbsp taco seasoning

Salt to taste

Directions:

1. Cut jalapeno in half lengthwise and remove seeds.
2. In a large mixing bowl, mix flour and eggs together, mix until smooth and lump free; set aside.
3. In another mixing bowl, combine cheddar cheese, taco seasoning and salt.
4. Place the bread crumbs in a shallow bowl.
5. Now spoon 2 tspful of cheese mixture into each jalapeño.
6. Dip each stuffed peppers into the egg batter and then into the bread crumbs.
7. Preheat air fryer to 400F.
8. Add the jalapenos to the preheated air fryer basket, and cook for 10 minutes until browned and crispy.

Vegan Burrito Bowl

Serving: 3   **Cooking time: 10 minutes**

Nutritional values

Calories 312 kcal

Fat 12.05 g

Total Carbs 48.77 g

Protein 11.43 g

Ingredients

8 corn tortillas

2 large egg plant, sliced

1 cup broccoli florets

1-1/4 cups, tin black beans, drained

1 large avocado, sliced

1 cup sweet corn

1 small head lettuce, chopped

1/4 cup cilantro, chopped

1 clove garlic, minced

1 tsp cumin

1 tsp chili powder

1 tsp paprika

1/2 tsp salt

For Salsa:

1 cup tomatoes, chopped

1 cup cucumber, chopped

1 tbsp lemon juice

Salt and black pepper to taste

For Garnishing:

Sour cream

Fresh parsley

Directions:

1. Season the eggplant and broccoli with garlic, cumin, chili powder, paprika and salt.
2. Preheat the air fryer to 400F.
3. Place the seasoned eggplant and broccoli in the air fryer.
4. Cook for about 10 minutes.

For Salsa:

5. In a small mixing bowl, combine all the salsa ingredients and set aside.

Assembling:

6. To assemble the vegan burrito bowl, place eggplant and broccoli into the bottom of the bowl.
7. Layer with black bean mixture.
8. Add avocado, sweet corn and cilantro.
9. Top with a spoonful of salsa and a dollop of sour cream.
10. Decorate the edges with the tortilla chips.
11. Top with shredded lettuce and parsley.

Eggplant Pizza

Serving: 6   **Cooking time: 15 minutes**

Nutritional values

Calories 201 kcal

Fat 8.26 g

Total Carbs 18.04 g

Protein 14.8 g

Ingredients

2 lbs. eggplant

1 cup pizza sauce

1 cup breadcrumbs

1 cup mozzarella cheese

1 cup cheddar cheese

1 large egg

1 tbsp taco seasoning

Directions:

1. Preheat the air fryer to 360F.
2. Cut eggplant into 1-inch thick disc.
3. In a mixing bowl, whisk egg until frothy.
4. In a medium shallow plate, combine breadcrumbs and taco seasoning.
5. Dip each eggplant slice into the egg and then into the breadcrumb mixture to coat evenly.
6. Now place a spoonful of pizza sauce.
7. Top with cheese.
8. Place the prepared eggplant in the air fryer basket.
9. Cook for 15 minutes until cheese is melted.

Veggie Stuffed Peppers

Serving: 6　　**Cooking time: 20 minutes**

Nutritional values

Calories 289 kcal　　Total Carbs 44.79 g

Fat 8.56 g　　Protein 10.47 g

Ingredients

6 green peppers

2 cups brown rice

1 cup tomatoes, chopped

1 cup corn

1 cup carrot, shredded

1 cup cabbage, shredded

1 cup cheddar cheese, shredded

1 tsp red chili powder

1 tsp chili sauce

1 tsp taco seasoning

Salt and pepper to taste

For Garnishing:

Fresh coriander leaves, chopped

Directions:

1. Cook rice according to the package.

2. Cut off each top of the peppers and scrape out the ribs and seeds, Set aside.

3. Preheat air fryer to 360F.

4. In a large mixing bowl, combine rice, tomatoes, corn, carrot, cabbage and chili sauce.

5. Season with red chili powder, taco seasoning, salt and pepper.

6. Stuff each pepper with the rice and vegetable mixture.

7. Sprinkle cheese on top and cook for 20 minutes.

8. When finished cooking; remove from the air fryer.

9. Garnish with fresh coriander leaves and serve.

Potato Croquettes

Serving: 8　　**Cooking time: 15 minutes**

Nutritional values

Calories 103 kcal　　Total Carbs 12.12 g

Fat 3.86 g　　Protein 5.03 g

Ingredients

2 large potatoes, boiled

1 cup peas

1/4 cup green onion, chopped

1/2 cup cheddar cheese

1 cup bread crumbs

2 large eggs

1 tsp onion powder

1 tsp garlic powder

1 tsp Worcestershire sauce

1 tsp vinegar

1/2 tsp black pepper

Salt to taste

Directions:

1. Mash the potatoes thoroughly.

2. Add peas, green onion, cheddar cheese, Worcestershire sauce, vinegar, black pepper and salt.

3. Shape the mixture into 15 croquettes.

4. In a mixing bowl, whisk eggs.

5. Place the bread crumbs, onion powder and garlic powder into a shallow bowl.

6. Dip each croquette into the egg and then into the bread crumbs mixture.

7. Grease the air fryer basket with some oil and preheat to 400F.

8. Place the croquettes into the prepared basket and cook for 15 minutes until nice golden brown.

9. Serve with your favorite dip.

Vegetable Lasagna

Serving: 4　　　**Cooking time: 25 minutes**

Nutritional values

Calories 1482 kcal

Fat 48.75 g

Total Carbs 194.41 g

Protein 81.75 g

Ingredients

14 lasagna noodles

2 large eggplants, sliced

1 large zucchini, sliced

1/2 cup onion, finely chopped

3 clove garlic, minced

1 cup pizza sauce

1 cup BBQ sauce

1 cup cheddar cheese

1 cup mozzarella cheese

Handful of basil leaves, chopped

1 tbsp Italian seasoning

1 tbsp olive oil

Salt and pepper to taste

Directions:

1. Cook lasagna noodles according to the package instructions.

2. In a frying pan, heat olive oil and sauté onion for 3 to 5 minutes, add garlic and fry for another 5 minutes.

3. Add eggplant and zucchini, season with Italian seasoning, salt and pepper; cook for 5 minutes.

4. Transfer the cooked veggies to a bowl and set aside.

5. Grease a 5-inch pan with some olive oil.

6. Place 3-4 lasagna sheets into the pan.

7. Add a layer of pizza sauce then cooked vegetables.

8. Top the layer with a spoonful of BBQ sauce.

9. Sprinkle cheese on top.

10. Repeat the layers until finished with all the ingredients.

11. Cover the pan with aluminum foil and place in the air fryer.

12. Cook for 15 minutes.

13. Garnish with basil; slice and serve hot.

Buffalo Cauliflower Wings

Serving: 8　　　**Cooking time: 10 minutes**

Nutritional values

BUFFALO WINGS:

Calories 48 kcal

Fat 0.32 g

Total Carbs 9.9 g

Protein 2.28 g

BUFFALO SAUCE:

Calories 59 kcal

Fat 0.11 g

Total Carbs 14.11 g

Protein 0.61 g

Ingredients

1 large head cauliflower

1/2 cup all-purpose flour

1/4 cup water

1 tsp paprika

1/4 tsp onion powder

1/4 tsp garlic powder

Salt to taste

For Buffalo Sauce:

1/2 cup tomato sauce

1/4 cup honey

3 tbsp soy sauce

1 tbsp apple cider vinegar

1 tsp paprika

1 tsp onion powder

1 tsp garlic powder

1/2 tsp cayenne powder

Directions:

1. Thoroughly wash the cauliflower and cut into bite-size pieces.

2. In a large mixing bowl, combine flour, water, paprika, onion powder, garlic powder and salt. Whisk until well combined.

3. Add cauliflower pieces to the batter, toss to coat evenly.

4. Preheat the air fryer to 400F.

5. Place the cauliflower in the air fryer basket.

6. Cook for 10 minutes, flipping the florets over half way through.

For Kebabs:

7. Meanwhile prepare the buffalo sauce.

8. Mix all the ingredients to a small serving bowl.

9. If desire, toss the baked cauliflower into the sauce or serve it separately.

Kale Chips

Serving: 6　　**Cooking time: 10 minutes**

Nutritional values

Calories 29 kcal

Fat 2.4 g

Total Carbs 1.65 g

Protein 0.68 g

Ingredients

5 cup kale leaves, stems removed and cut into 1-inch pieces 1 tsp garlic powder

1/2 tsp paprika

1 tbsp olive oil

Salt

Directions:

1. Preheat the air fryer to 360F.

2. In a large mixing bowl, combine kale and oil.

3. Season with garlic powder and paprika; toss until thoroughly coated.

4. Transfer the kale leaves to the air fryer basket and cook for 8-10 minutes.

5. Once the chips are done, immediately transfer to a baking sheet, lined with parchment paper; let it cool for about 10 minutes.

6. Sprinkle salt and serve.

Vegetable Spring Rolls

Serving: 8　　**Cooking time: 15 minutes**

Nutritional values

Calories 113 kcal

Fat 1.13 g

Total Carbs 21.63 g

Protein 4.03 g

Ingredients

8 Spring roll wrappers

1 cup cabbage, shredded

1 cup carrot, shredded

1 cup green bell pepper, sliced

2 clove garlic, minced

1 egg, beaten

1 tsp Worcestershire sauce

1 tsp vinegar

1 tsp oil

1 tsp black pepper

Salt to taste

Directions:

1. Heat a large non-stick wok over medium-high heat.

2. Add oil and heat until shimmering.

3. Add garlic and sauté for 3 minutes.

4. Add cabbage, carrot and bell pepper; cook for 5-7 minutes.

5. Stir in the vinegar and Worcestershire sauce, let cool at room temperature.

6. Season with salt and pepper.

7. Place a single roll wrapper on a clean surface.

8. Place a tbsp full of vegetable mixture in the center of the wrapper.

9. Brush the edges with egg.

10. Roll up tightly with ends tucked inside.

11. Preheat the air fryer to 400F and brush the basket with some oil.

12.

Cheesy Zucchini Boats

Serving: 4   **Cooking time: 15 minutes**

Nutritional values

Calories 235 kcal

Fat 10.82 g

Total Carbs 17.26 g

Protein 20.93 g

Ingredients

4 large zucchini

1 cup mozzarella cheese, shredded

1 cup cheddar cheese, shredded

2 clove garlic, minced

1 cup salsa

1 tsp onion powder

1 tsp chili powder

1 tsp oregano

Salt to taste

Directions:

1. Preheat air fryer to 400F.
2. Cut the zucchini in half lengthwise.
3. Scoop out the inside of zucchini with a melon scooper and chop them into cubes.
4. In a mixing bowl, combine zucchini, salsa, garlic, onion powder, chili powder, oregano and salt.
5. Place the mixture back to the prepared zucchini boats.
6. Sprinkle with cheddar and mozzarella cheese.
7. Place the zucchini boats in the air fryer.
8. Cook for 15 minutes until cheese is melted.

Vegetable Sushi

Serving: 4   **Cooking time: 10 minutes**

Nutritional values

Calories 497 kcal

Fat 13.17 g

Total Carbs 85.5 g

Protein 8.04 g

Ingredients

5 sheets of sushi nori

2 cup rice

1 cup avocado, sliced

1/2 cup carrots, shredded

1/4 cup mayonnaise

1 tsp garlic powder

1 tsp onion powder

1 tsp soy sauce

1 tsp sesame oil

For Coating:

1/2 cup breadcrumbs

For Serving:

Soy sauce

Directions:

1. Preheat air fryer to 400F.
2. In a mixing bowl, combine avocado, carrots, garlic powder, onion powder and soy sauce.
3. Lay a nori sheet on a dry surface, shiny side down.
4. Pat rice on top of the nori sheet, about 1-inch thick layer.
5. Place avocado and carrots mixture over the rice.
6. Spread a spoonful of mayonnaise.
7. Starting from the one end with the filling, tightly roll up your sushi.
8. Place the breadcrumbs into a shallow bowl.
9. Grab a sushi roll, dip in soy sauce & then in the breadcrumbs.
10. Make sure to coat evenly. Repeat until finished with the rest of the rolls.
11. Brush the air fryer basket with sesame oil.
12.

13. Slice the sushi rolls into pieces and enjoy with soy sauce.

Tofu Satay

Serving: 6   **Cooking time: 15 minutes**

Nutritional values

FOR TOFU SATAY:
Calories 176 kcal
Fat 11.3 g
Total Carbs 6.39 g
Protein 16.08 g

FOR SAUCE:
Calories 73 kcal
Fat 3.91 g
Total Carbs 8.33 g
Protein 1.59 g

Ingredients

2 Blocks extra-firm tofu

2 tbsp sesame seeds

For Marinade:

3 tbsp soy sauce

1 tsp peanut sauce

1 tbsp peanut butter

1 tsp garlic powder

For Peanut Sauce:

1/2 cup peanut butter

1 tsp Dijon mustard

1/2 tsp chili flakes

1 tbsp honey

Directions:

1. Preheat air fryer to 380F.

2. Start by preparing a marinade by mixing, soy sauce, peanut sauce, peanut butter and garlic powder.

3. Cut tofu into cubes.

4. Dunk the tofu into the marinade and thread 3 cubes onto skewers.

5. Sprinkle sesame seeds.

6. Place the skewers in the air fryer basket.

7. Cook for 15 minutes, turning occasionally until evenly browned.

8. While the tofu is cooking prepare the peanut sauce.

9. In a small serving bowl, combine all the sauce ingredients; mix until well combined.

10. Once the tofu is done, serve hot with the sauce.

Classic Falafel

Serving: 5   **Cooking time: 10 minutes**

Nutritional values

Calories 224 kcal

Fat 5.81 g

Total Carbs 33.7 g

Protein 10.37 g

Ingredients

2 can chick peas, rinsed and drained

1 small onion, chopped

1/4 cup parsley

1 cup bread crumbs

1 large egg

2 clove garlic, minced

3 tbsp all-purpose flour

1 tsp cumin

1 tbsp sesame seeds

1 tsp olive oil

1 tsp black pepper

Salt to taste

Directions:

1. Add chickpeas, parsley, garlic, flour, cumin, black pepper and salt to a food processor, pulse until well combined.

2. Transfer the mixture to a bowl, add onion and sesame seeds; mix well.

3. Make small balls and flatten with the help of your palm to form a Pattie shape.

4. Place the bread crumbs into a shallow bowl.

5. Whisk egg in a bowl.

6. Dip each Pattie into the egg and then into bread crumbs.

7. Grease the air fryer basket with oil and preheat to 360F for 10 minutes.

8. Place the patties in the air fryer basket.

9. Cook for 20 minutes; flipping when one side is deep golden brown.

Vegan Tacos

Serving: 6　　**Cooking time: 10 minutes**

Nutritional values

Calories 368 kcal

Fat 14.24 g

Total Carbs 50.97 g

Protein 10.83 g

Ingredients

2 cups broccoli florets

2 cup cauliflower florets;
cut into bite-sized pieces

1 cup red bell pepper, sliced

1 can chickpeas, drained
and rinsed

1 tbsp taco seasoning

1 tbsp oil

For Filling:

8 small tortillas shell

1 cup red cabbage,
chopped

1 large avocado, sliced

1/2 cup sour cream

For Garnishing:

1/4 cup fresh cilantro
leaves, chopped

1/4 tsp paprika

Directions:

1. Preheat the air fryer to 400F.

2. In a large mixing bowl, add broccoli, cauliflower, bell pepper and chickpeas.

3. Add taco seasoning and oil; toss until well combined.

4. Place the veggies into the air fryer basket and cook for 10 minutes; shaking the basket occasionally.

5. Place the cabbage, avocado, and cooked veggies in taco shells.

6. Top with a dollop of sour cream.

7. Sprinkle some paprika on top and garnish with fresh cilantro.

Sweet and Sour Cauliflower Stir Fry

Serving: 4　　**Cooking time: 20 minutes**

Nutritional values

Calories 83 kcal

Fat 0.63 g

Total Carbs 18.29 g

Protein 4.38 g

Ingredients

1 large head
cauliflower, cut into
florets

1/2 cup onion, sliced

2 clove garlic, minced

1 tbsp tamarind paste

1 tbsp honey

1 tbsp Worcestershire sauce

Salt and pepper to taste

For Coating:

Green onion, sliced

Directions:

1. Preheat air fryer to 360F.

2. Mix all the ingredients to a bowl, toss until well combined.

3. Dump everything into the air fryer basket and cook for 20 minutes, shaking the basket occasionally.

4. Garnish with sliced green onion and serve with your favorite dip.

Vegetable Fritters

Serving: 6   **Cooking time: 15 minutes**

Nutritional values

Calories 105 kcal   Total Carbs 22.21 g

Fat 0.78 g   Protein 3.24 g

Ingredients

1 cup corn kernels   1 tsp garlic powder

1 cup carrots, shredded   1 tsp paprika

1 cup spinach, chopped   1 tsp oregano

1 cup potatoes, cubed   1 tsp thyme

1/2 cup cornmeal powder   1 tsp black pepper

1 large egg   Salt to taste

1 tsp onion powder

Directions:

1. In a large mixing bowl, combine corn, carrots, spinach and potatoes.

2. Add onion powder, garlic powder, paprika, oregano, thyme, black pepper and salt.

3. Add cornmeal powder and crack the egg.

4. Mix until well combined.

5. Preheat air fryer to 400F.

6. Grease the air fryer basket with some oil.

7. Using an ice cream scooper, drop a scoopful of batter into the basket.

8. Cook for about 15 minutes, flipping after every 5 minutes to make sure fritters are evenly browned.

Sweet Potato Jackets

Serving: 5   **Cooking time: 25 minutes**

Nutritional values

Calories 253 kcal   Total Carbs 23.73 g

Fat 14.59 g   Protein 7.95 g

Ingredients

3 large sweet potatoes   For Garnishing:

1/3 cup sweet corns   1 tbsp chives, sliced

1/4 cup green onion, sliced

1/2 cup mayonnaise

1/2 cup sour cream

1 cup cheddar cheese

1 tsp hot chili sauce

1 tsp black pepper

Salt to taste

Directions:

1. Cut a cross on top of each sweet potato.

2. Preheat the air fryer to 390F.

3. Sprinkle some salt and cook for 20 minutes.

4. Once the potatoes are done, remove from the air fryer.

5. Using a tbsp, carefully scoop out the flesh from potatoes, leaving the skin unbroken.

6. Place the flesh and the remaining ingredients to a bowl; mix until well combined.

7. Scoop back the mixture into the potato skin.

8. Sprinkle with some more cheese.

9. Place the jackets back to the air fryer and cook for additional 5 minutes.

10.

Sticky BBQ Tofu

Serving: 4   **Cooking time: 10 minutes**

Nutritional values

Calories 231 kcal

Fat 6.88 g

Total Carbs 34.69 g

Protein 11.67 g

Ingredients

1 Block extra-firm tofu

1/2 cup BBQ sauce

1/4 cup honey

1 tsp black pepper

For Garnishing:

1/2 cup Parsley, chopped

Directions:

1. Cut the tofu in cubes.

2. In a plastic storage bag, add BBQ sauce, honey and black pepper, shake until well combined.

3. Add cubed tofu and shake, let marinate for half an hour.

4. Preheat the air fryer to 360F.

5. Place the tofu in the air fryer, one layer at a time.

6. Cook for 10 minutes.

7. Garnish with parsley and serve.

Black Bean Burger

Serving: 6   **Cooking time: 20 minutes**

Nutritional values

Calories 101 kcal

Fat 0.64 g

Total Carbs 18.63 g

Protein 5.96 g

Ingredients

2 cups black bean, drained and rinsed

1/2 cup onion, finely chopped

2 slices bread, crumbled

1/4 cup cilantro

1 tbsp lemon juice

1 tsp cumin

1 tsp garlic powder

1 tsp oregano

Salt to taste

For Serving:

6 Hamburger buns

1 cup mayonnaise

1 avocado, sliced

1 large tomato, sliced

Lettuce, shredded

Directions:

1. In a food processor, except onion pulse all the ingredient together until well combined.
2. Using the palm of your hand shape the mixture into 6 patties.
3. If they crack just press the mixture gently back together.
4. Preheat air fryer to 400F.
5. Place the patties into the air fryer and cook for about 20 minutes.
6. Allow to cook on one side until golden, flip and continue cooking the other side.
7. Spread a spoonful of mayonnaise onto the bun.
8. Place a Pattie on top.
9. Add avocado and lettuce.
10. Top with a slice of tomato
11. Cover with the second bun and serve.

Desserts

Chocolate Fudge Brownies

Serving: 6 **Cooking time: 20 minutes**

Nutritional values

Calories 363 kcal

Fat 23.87 g

Total Carbs 35.86 g

Protein 4.45 g

Ingredients

1 cup flour

1 cup sugar

3/4 cup butter

1/3 cup cocoa powder

1 tsp baking powder

2 eggs

1 tsp vanilla extract

1/4 tsp salt

For Serving:

Vanilla ice cream

Directions:

1. Preheat the air fryer to 350F and grease a baking tin with non-stick spray.

2. In a mixing bowl, sift together flour, cocoa powder, baking powder and salt; set aside.

3. In another mixing bowl, beat butter, sugar and vanilla extract together, beat until light and fluffy.

4. Add eggs and whisk again until pale and creamy.

5. Now fold in the dry ingredients and mix until well combined.

6. Pour the batter into the prepared pan.

7. Set the pan in the air fryer basket and bake for 20 minutes or until toothpick inserted out comes clean.

8. Top with vanilla ice cream and serve.

Coconut Cookies

Serving: 8 **Cooking time: 15 minutes**

Nutritional values

Calories 243 kcal

Fat 13.9 g

Total Carbs 27.64 g

Protein 2.44 g

Ingredients

1 cup flour

3/4 cup sugar

3/4 cup coconut, shredded

1/2 cup butter

1 tsp baking powder

2 tbsp cornstarch

1 large egg

1 tsp coconut or vanilla extract

Directions:

1. In a mixing bowl, beat butter & sugar until light & fluffy.

2. Add eggs and coconut extract, beat again.

3. In another mixing bowl, combine flour, cornstarch and baking powder together.

4. Add dry ingredients and continue beating until mixture turns into a dough.

5. Fold in the shredded coconut.

6. Wrap the dough into a plastic wrap and refrigerate for at least 2 hours.

7. Form 1-inch balls and place on to a large serving plate.

8. Slightly flatten the balls with the back of the spoon.

9. Line the air fryer basket with parchment paper and preheat the air fryer to 360F.

10. Carefully place the cookies in the basket with a little gap in between each other.

11. Cook for about 15 minutes until slightly golden brown.

Chocolate Soufflé

Serving: 4   **Cooking time: 15 minutes**

Nutritional values

Calories 350 kcal

Fat 24.31 g

Total Carbs 27.31 g

Protein 6.7 g

Ingredients

3/4 cup chocolate chips

1/4 cup butter

3 large eggs, separated

4 tbsp sugar

2 tbsp cocoa powder

1 tsp vanilla extract

2 tbsp powdered sugar, for dusting

Directions:

1. Preheat air fryer to 400F and lightly butter 4 ramekin dishes.

2. Melt chocolate chips and butter together, either in the microwave or in a double boiler.

3. Remove from heat and let cool to room temperature, about 10 minutes.

4. Stir in the egg yolks, sugar, cocoa powder and vanilla extract; mix until well combined.

5. In a separated large bowl, using an electric mixer beat egg whites until soft peaks are formed.

6. Fold the whites into the yolk mixture.

7. Transfer the batter carefully to the buttered ramekins, taking care not to get on top edge of the ramekins.

8. Now carefully place the ramekins in the air fryer and bake for 15 minutes until puffed.

9. Dust with powdered sugar and serve immediately.

Assorted Donuts

Serving: 8   **Cooking time: 10 minutes**

Nutritional values

Calories 196 kcal

Fat 7.84 g

Total Carbs 27.62 g

Protein 3.62 g

Ingredients

For Donuts:
2 cups all-purpose flour
5 tbsp butter, cold cut into cubes
1/3 cup milk
3 tbsp sugar
1 tsp baking powder
For Topping:
1 cup melted Chocolate

For Glaze:
1 cup powdered sugar
Pink food coloring
3 drops vanilla extract
3 tbsp water
For Cinnamon Sugar:
1/2 cup powdered sugar
1 tsp cinnamon

Directions:

For Glaze:

1. Mix powdered sugar, food color, vanilla extract and water to a bowl; mix until thick paste consistency.

For Cinnamon Sugar:

2. Mix cinnamon and sugar together in a bowl & set aside.

For Donuts:

3. In a large mixing bowl, combine flour, sugar and baking powder.

4. Add the cubed butter, using your fingers crumble the mixture.

5. Add milk and knead until dough comes together.

6. Transfer the mixture onto a lightly floured surface and knead until dough is no more-sticky.

7. Wrap the dough in a plastic wrap and refrigerate for at least 30 minutes to set.

8. Roll the dough into a 1/8 inch-thick rectangle.

9. Using a donut cutter cut circles out of the dough.

10. Preheat air fryer to 400F and lightly butter the air fryer basket with some oil.

11. Place the 4 donuts in the air fryer at a time, spacing evenly to avoid touching.

12. Cook for 10 minutes until browned and puffed.

13. Once the donuts are browned, immediately roll some donuts into the cinnamon sugar mixture.

14. Dip some into the glaze and chocolate sauce.

15. Place on a wire rack to cool.

16. Serve and enjoy.

Chocolate Cake

Serving: 10   **Cooking time: 30 minutes**

Nutritional values

Calories 221 kcal   Total Carbs 19.28 g

Fat 15.34 g   Protein 2.99 g

Ingredients

1-1/2 cup all-purpose flour
1 cup sugar
3/4 cup butter
2 large eggs
1/4 cup cocoa powder
1/4 cup milk
1 tsp baking powder
1/2 tsp baking soda
1 tbsp coffee powder
1 tsp vanilla extract

For Buttercream Frosting:
1-1/2 cup powdered sugar
3/4 cup butter, softened
1/4 cup cocoa powder
2 tsp coffee powder
1 tsp vanilla extract
For Garnishing:
1/2 cup Glazed cherries

Directions:

1. Preheat air fryer to 360F and grease a baking tin with non-stick spray.
2. In a large bowl, beat sugar and butter until smooth and creamy.
3. Add eggs, milk and vanilla extract; beat again until pale and fluffy.
4. Sift flour, cocoa, baking powder, baking soda and coffee into a large bowl, whisk briefly to combine.
5. Fold the dry ingredients into the wet mixture; mix until well combined and lump free.
6. Pour the batter into the prepared pan and bake for about 30 minutes or until knife inserted into the center comes out clean.
7. Once the cake is done, remove from the air fryer and turn out onto a wire rack to cool completely.

For Buttercream Frosting:

8. Using an electric mixer, beat butter, sugar and vanilla extract together in a bowl.
9. Sift in cocoa and coffee powder, beat until smooth and creamy.

Frosting:

10. Cut the cake into two equal halves.
11. Sandwich the layers together with buttercream, then spread the rest on top.
12. Place the cake in refrigerator for 20 minutes.
13. Top with some cherries, slice and serve.

Pineapple Bites

Serving: 6   **Cooking time: 5 minutes**

Nutritional values

Calories 223 kcal   Total Carbs 31.98 g

Fat 7.63 g   Protein 6.58 g

Ingredients

8 won ton wrappers

1 small egg

For Filling:

1 cup pineapple, chopped

1/2 cup cream cheese

1/4 cup raisins

1 tsp butter

Directions:

1. Mix together all the filling ingredients to a bowl and set aside.

2. Place a tsp full of pineapple filling in center of won ton wrapper.

3. Brush the edges with egg, and fold all the 4 edges together to seal tightly.

4. Preheat air fryer to 400F and grease the basket with non-stick spray.

5. Cook for 5 minutes or until golden and crispy.

Cinnamon Sugar Churros

Serving: 4   **Cooking time: 10 minutes**

Nutritional values

Calories 344 kcal

Fat 23.35g

Total Carbs 28.11 g

Protein 5.27 g

Ingredients

1 cup all-purpose flour

2 tbsp sugar

1/2 cup butter

2 eggs

1 cup water

1 tsp vanilla extract

For Cinnamon Sugar Coating:

1 cup powdered sugar

1 tsp cinnamon

For Serving:

Chocolate sauce

Directions:

1. Preheat the air fryer at 360F while you make the churros batter.
2. In a mixing bowl, whisk together eggs and vanilla extract.
3. In a medium saucepan over medium-high heat, heat butter, sugar and water; bring to boil.
4. Immediately stir in the flour and mix vigorously until well blended.
5. Remove from the heat and let it cool at room temperature.
6. Pour the beaten egg and mix again vigorously using a wooden spoon.
7. Place the dough into a piping bag fitted with star piping tip.
8. Pipe 6-inch long churros to a parchment lined baking sheet.
9. Refrigerate for 15 minutes to set the dough.
10. Place the churros into the preheated air fryer and cook for 10 minutes.
11. Meanwhile mix the cinnamon and powdered sugar into a mixing bowl.
12. Once the churros are done, roll them in the cinnamon sugar mixture.
13. cool at room temperature.
14. Serve with chocolate sauce.

Raisin Bread Pudding with Chocolate Sauce

Serving: 6   **Cooking time: 15 minutes**

Nutritional values

Calories 239 kcal

Fat 11.37 g

Total Carbs 27.73 g

Protein 6.45 g

Ingredients

5 cups bread slices, cubed

2 cups milk

2 eggs

1/4 cup brown sugar

1/4 cup butter, melted

3 tbsp raisins

1/4 tsp nutmeg

1 tsp vanilla extract

For Chocolate Sauce:

1 cup chocolate chips

3 tbsp cream

1 tsp vanilla extract

Directions:

For Sauce:

1. mbine all the sauce ingredients to a bowl and microwave for 2 minutes.
2. frigerate the sauce while the pudding is cooking.

For Pudding:

3. eheat the air fryer at 360F and grease a baking pan with some butter.
4. a large mixing bowl, whisk beat eggs.
5. d milk, sugar, butter, nutmeg and vanilla extract; whisk again.
6. d bread cubes and raisins; stir gently.
7. ur the mixture into the prepared pan and cook for 15 minutes, until top is golden brown and a knife inserted in the center comes out clean.
8. izzle chocolate sauce on top and serve.

Blueberry Cheesecake

Serving: 8   **Cooking time: 30 minutes**

Nutritional values

Calories 345 kcal

Fat 20.75 g

Total Carbs 35.79 g

Protein 6.39 g

Ingredients

For Crust:

1 cup graham cracker, finely crushed

1/4 cup butter, melted

For Blueberry Sauce:

2 cups blue berries

1/4 cup water

1 tbsp cornstarch

1 tsp lemon juice

For Filling:

2 cup blueberries

1-1/2 cup cream cheese

1/4 cup powdered sugar

3 eggs

2 tbsp all-purpose flour

1 tsp lemon zest

Directions:

For Crust:

1. mbine the crust ingredients in a small bowl and press the mixture into the bottom of the springform cake pan.

For Cheesecake:

2. eheat the air fryer to 360F.

3. a large mixing bowl, beat cream cheese, sugar, flour and lemon zest; beat until smooth and creamy.

4. d eggs one at a time, mix until well combined.

5. ntly stir in the blueberries.

6. ur the batter evenly over the top of the crust, cover the pan with aluminum foil.

7. ace the pan in the air fryer and cook for 20 minutes.

For Sauce:

8. a saucepan combine blueberries, water and cornstarch.

9. d lemon juice and let simmer for about 10 minutes until sauce is thickened.

10. h the blueberries with a fork.

11. e the cheesecake is done, remove from the fryer and let cool at room temperature.

12. the cheesecake with blueberry sauce.

13. rigerate for 30 minutes. 14.

Dish out the cake and enjoy.

Tropical Egg Rolls

Serving: 6   **Cooking time: 10 minutes**

◇◇

Nutritional values

Calories 217 kcal

Fat 6.5 g

Total Carbs 34.07 g

Protein 5.95 g

◇◇

Ingredients

8 egg roll wrappers

For Filling:

1 cup apple, chopped

1 cup strawberries cut into chunks

1/2 cup pineapple, chopped

1/2 cup cream cheese

1 tsp lemon juice

1 tsp cinnamon

For Serving:

1 cup whipped cream

◇◇

Directions:

1. Preheat the air fryer to 360F and grease the basket with some oil.

2. In a medium sized mixing bowl beat cream cheese, lemon juice and cinnamon until well combined. Gently fold in the chopped fruits; set aside.

3. Lay an egg roll wrapper down on a floured surface, add a spoonful of filling in the center of each wrapper and wet the edges with water.

4. Roll tightly with ends tucked inside.

5. Place the stuffed rolls carefully in the air fryer and cook for 10 minutes, turning over once halfway through until nice golden brown.

6. Serve warm with whipped cream.

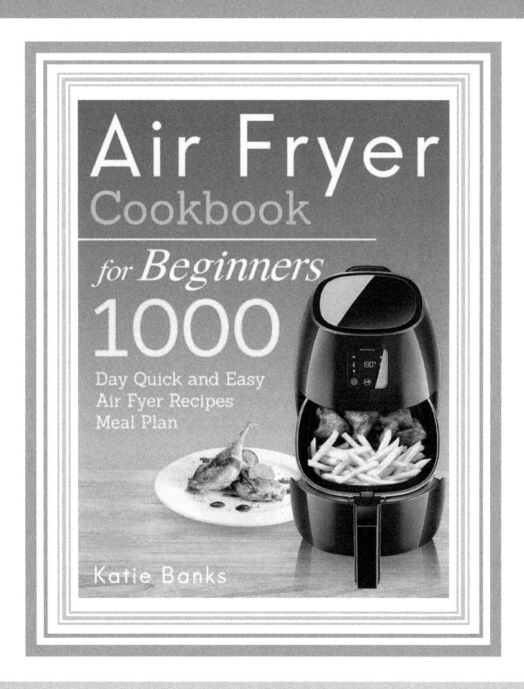

Korean Chicken Wings

Serving: 2 **Cooking Time: 20 minutes**

Nutritional values

Calories 350 kcal

Fat 8.27 g

Total Carbs 14.89 g

Protein 50.46 g

Ingredients

1 lb. chicken wings

1/4 cup BBQ sauce

1 tbsp soy sauce

1/4 tsp black pepper

For Garnishing:

1/4 cup cilantro, chopped

Directions:

1. Add all the ingredients to the chicken wings and let marinate for an hour.
2. Preheat the air fryer to 380F.
3. Transfer the chicken wings into the air fryer basket.
4. Cook for 20 minutes at 400F until crisp and lightly browned.
5. Transfer to a serving bowl, sprinkle chopped cilantro and serve.

Honey Drumsticks with Citrus

Serving: 2 **Cooking Time: 15 minutes**

Nutritional values

Calories 783 kcal

Fat 40.02 g

Total Carbs 50.05 g

Protein 56.01 g

Ingredients

1 1/3 lb. chicken drumsticks

1/3 cup honey

2 tbsp teriyaki sauce

2/3 tbsp butter

1 tbsp lemon juice

2 tsp olive oil

For Garnishing:

1/2 cup parsley, finely chopped

Lemon wedges

Directions:

1. Preheat the air fryer to 360F.
2. Use an oil brush, to coat the drumsticks very lightly with olive oil.
3. Place the drumsticks in the air fryer basket.
4. Cook for 15 minutes, turning the drumsticks halfway after few minutes with a tong.
5. Meanwhile combine all the remaining ingredients to a bowl and microwave for 3 minutes.
6. When the drumsticks are cooked through, brush them with the prepared sauce until well coated.
7. Garnish with chopped parsley and serve hot with lemon wedges.

IndianTandoori Chicken

Serving: 2   **Cooking Time: 25 minutes**

Nutritional values

Calories 311 kcal   Total Carbs 5.87 g

Fat 8.89 g   Protein 49.26 g

Ingredients

1lb. chicken

2/3 cup yogurt

1 tsp ginger

1 tsp garlic paste

1 tsp turmeric

1 tsp red chili powder

1 tsp ground cumin

1 1/2 tbsp lemon juice

For Garnishing:

1/3 cup onion, sliced into rings

2 lemon wedges

Directions:

1. Start by preparing a marinade, in a large mixing bowl, combine yogurt, ginger garlic paste, turmeric, chili powder, cumin and lemon juice; mix until well combined.

2. Rinse the chicken and pat the excess moisture with paper towel.

3. With the help of a sharp knife, mark the slits in the center of each chicken.

4. Pour the marinade over the chicken and let marinate for 2 hours.

5. Line the air fryer basket with aluminum foil.

6. Preheat the air fryer to 360F.

7. Place the chicken into the basket and cook for 25 minutes at 380F.

8. Once the chicken is done, transfer the chicken to a serving dish.

9. Top with onion rings and serve with lemon wedges.

Curry Roasted Chicken

Serving: 2   **Cooking Time: 30 minutes**

Nutritional values

Calories 392 kcal   Total Carbs 3.53 g

Fat 12.99 g   Protein 62.22 g

Ingredients

1 1/3 lb. whole chicken

2 tsp olive oil

For Dry Rub:

1 tsp garlic powder

1 tsp onion powder

1 tsp paprika

1 tsp curry powder

Salt and pepper to taste

Directions:

1. Preheat the air fryer to 360F for 10 minutes.

2. Thoroughly wash the chicken, remove the neck and giblets.

3. Pat the excess moisture with paper towel.

4. With the help of a sharp knife, mark the slits in the middle of the chicken.

5. Brush the chicken with oil; set aside.

6. In a large mixing bowl, mix all the spices together.

7. Generously rub the spices onto each side of the chicken.

8. Place the chicken into the air fryer basket.

9. Cook at 400F for about 15 minutes.

10. Turn the chicken upside down and cook for another 15 minutes at 360F.

11. Once the chicken is done cooking, transfer it to a large serving dish.

12. Let rest for 10 minutes at room temperature, slice and serve.

Honey & Thyme Glazed Turkey

Serving: 2 **Cooking time: 20 minutes**

Nutritional values

Calories 670 kcal

Fat 18.97 g

Total Carbs 12.91 g

Protein 107.56 g

Ingredients

2 lb. whole turkey

2 tbsp butter

2 tbsp honey

1 tsp rosemary

1 tsp thyme

1 tsp oregano

1/2 tsp paprika

1 tsp black pepper

1 tbsp olive oil

Salt to taste

Directions:

1. Preheat air fryer to 400F.
2. Brush the olive oil all over the turkey.
3. In a small bowl, combine butter, honey, rosemary, thyme, oregano, paprika, black pepper and salt; rub the mixture generously all over the turkey.
4. Place the turkey into the air fryer basket and cook for 20 minutes or until the final temperature of turkey reads 165F.
5. Flip the turkey upside down after 10 minutes.
6. Remove the turkey and let rest for 10 minutes before serving.

Turkish Kabobs

Serving: 2 **Cooking time: 30 minutes**

Nutritional values

Calories 283 kcal

Fat 18.24 g

Total Carbs 13.77 g

Protein 15.91 g

Ingredients

½ lb. turkey, boneless & cubed

½ cups pineapple, diced

½ medium onion, cubed

½ cup green bell pepper, cubed

For Marinade:

½ cup pineapple juice

1 clove garlic, minced

1 tsp ginger

1 tbsp Worcestershire sauce

1 tbsp vinegar

Salt and black pepper to taste

2 wooden skewers

Directions:

1. Start by preparing a marinade; pour all the ingredients into a large mixing bowl.
2. Add turkey and marinate for 3 hours.
3. Spray the air fryer basket with some cooking spray and preheat at 400F.
4. Alternately thread turkey, pineapple, onion and bell pepper onto the skewers.
5. Place the skewers into the prepared basket and cook for about 30 minutes or until turkey temperature reaches 165F.

Lemon Garlic Turkey

Serving: 2   **Cooking time: 25 minutes**

Nutritional values

Calories 267 kcal

Fat 12.96 g

Total Carbs 2.47 g

Protein 33.47 g

Ingredients

2/3 lb. turkey breast, with skin

1/3 cup cherry tomatoes

2/3 clove garlic, minced

2 tbsp + 2 tsp fresh lemon juice

2 tsp lemon peel, grated

1 tsp oregano

1 tsp thyme

1 tbsp olive oil

Salt to taste

For Garnishing:

Lemon, sliced

Directions:

1. Thoroughly wash the turkey breast and pat the excess moisture with paper towel.

2. Grease the air fryer basket with olive oil and preheat at 360F.

3. In a small mixing bowl, mix garlic, lemon juice, lemon peel, oregano, thyme and salt.

4. Generously rub the mixture all over the turkey breast.

5. Place the turkey breast and cherry tomatoes into the prepared air fryer basket.

6. Cook for 25 minutes.

7. Garnish with some sliced lemon and serve hot.

Avocado Turkey Salad Patties

Serving: 2   **Cooking time: 20 minutes**

Nutritional values

Calories 302 kcal

Fat 26.49 g

Total Carbs 3.02 g

Protein 12.13 g

Ingredients

¼ lb. ground turkey

2 tbsp breadcrumbs

2 tbsp green onion, chopped

2 tbsp onion, chopped

1 clove garlic, minced

1 large egg

1 tbsp teriyaki sauce

1/2 tsp oil

Salt and pepper to taste

For Avocado Salad:

1/2 small avocado, diced

1/4 cup cherry tomato

2 tbsp onion, chopped

Salt and black pepper to taste

Directions:

1. In a large mixing bowl mix all the ingredients together.

2. Shape the mixture into 8 patties, 1/2 inch thick.

3. Preheat the air fryer to 400F.

4. Place the patties into the air fryer basket and cook for 20 minutes.

5. Meanwhile mix all the salad ingredients to a serving bowl and set aside.

6. Serve the patties with avocado salad.

Creamy Pork Chops

Serving: 2 **Cooking time: 15 minutes**

Nutritional values

Calories 310 kcal

Fat 15.37 g

Total Carbs 1.74 g

Protein 39.56 g

Ingredients

2 bone-in pork chops

2 clove garlic, minced

1 tbsp oregano

1 tsp paprika

1 tsp black pepper

1 1/2 tbsp butter

Salt to taste

For Garnishing:

¼ cup green onion, chopped

Directions:

1. Preheat the air fryer to 400F for 8 minutes.

2. In a mixing bowl, combine butter, garlic, oregano, paprika, black pepper, salt.

3. Coat the pork chop with the rub.

4. Place the pork chops into the air fryer basket and cook for 15 minutes, flipping half way through.

5. Garnish with green onion and serve.

Coleslaw Pulled Pork BBQ Style

Serving: 2 **Cooking time: 20 minutes**

Nutritional values

Calories 429 kcal

Fat 18.01 g

Total Carbs 21.02 g

Protein 43.23 g

Ingredients

1 lb. pork shoulder

For Coleslaw:

1/3 cup mayonnaise

1/3 cup cabbage, shredded

2 ½ tbsp carrots, shredded

1/2 tsp sugar

Salt and black pepper to taste

For Rub:

1/3 cup BBQ sauce

1/2 tsp garlic powder

1 tsp chili powder

1 tsp paprika

1/4 tsp cinnamon powder

1 1/2 tbsp olive oil

1 tsp black pepper

1 tsp salt

Directions:

For Coleslaw:

1. Mix all the coleslaw ingredients to a small serving bowl and set aside.

For Rub:

2. In a large mixing bowl, combine all the rub ingredients.

3. Add pork and marinate for 3 hours.

4. Preheat the air fryer to 400F.

5. Place the pork in the air fryer basket.

6. Pour the remaining sauce over the top of the pork.

7. Cook for 20 minutes or until internal temperature read 160F.

8. Flip the pork at the halfway cooking point.

9. Once the pork is cooked through, shred it using two forks to "pull" it apart.

10.

Crusty Rosemary Pork Ribs

Serving: 2   **Cooking time: 25 minutes**

Nutritional values

Calories 838 kcal

Fat 32.41 g

Total Carbs 7.94 g

Protein 119.87 g

Ingredients

2 ½ lbs. pork ribs, baby back or spare ribs

1/2 cup bread crumbs

1 small egg

1 tbsp Worcestershire sauce

1 tsp onion powder

1 tsp garlic powder

1 tsp thyme

1 tsp rosemary

1 tsp black pepper

Salt to taste

Directions:

1. Season the pork with salt and black pepper.
2. Place the bread crumbs into a shallow bowl.
3. Add onion powder, garlic powder, thyme, rosemary, black pepper and salt, mix until well combine.
4. Whisk egg and Worcestershire sauce in another bowl.
5. Grab a rib, dunk in the egg and then into the bread crumb mixture.
6. Pat with your hands until they're fully coated.
7. Preheat the air fryer to 400F.
8. Grease the air fryer basket with some oil.
9. Place the ribs into the basket and cook for 25 minutes.
10. Transfer the ribs to a serving plate and serve with your favorite dip.

Pork Tenderloin in Balsamic Vinegar

Serving: 2   **Cooking time: 20 minutes**

Nutritional values

Calories 519 kcal

Fat 11.96 g

Total Carbs 6.34 g

Protein 89.35 g

Ingredients

1 ½ lbs. pork tenderloin, cut into four pieces

¼ cup balsamic vinegar

1 clove garlic, minced

1 tsp oregano

Salt to taste

For Garnishing:

Basil leaves

Directions:

1. Start by preparing a marinade, in a large mixing bowl, combine balsamic vinegar, garlic, oregano and salt.
2. Add the pork pieces and let sit in refrigerator for at least an hour.
3. Preheat the air fryer to 360F.
4. Place the marinated pork into the air fryer basket and cook for 20 minutes.
5. Top with some basil leaves and serve.

Japanese Filet Mignon

Serving: 2 **Cooking time: 20 minutes**

Nutritional values

Calories 907 kcal

Fat 71.81 g

Total Carbs 3.19 g

Protein 62.69 g

Ingredients

1 1/2 large beef ribeye or filet mignon steaks

1 cup broccoli florets

2 cloves garlic, minced

1 tbsp teriyaki sauce

1/2 tbsp Worcestershire sauce

1 tsp oregano

Salt to taste

Directions:

1. In a small mixing bowl, combine garlic, teriyaki sauce, Worcestershire sauce, oregano and salt.

2. Pour the marinade over the steak, turn upside down to coat well.

3. Cover and refrigerate for at least 6 hours.

4. Preheat the air fryer to 400F and grease the basket with some oil.

5. Place the steaks in the air fryer and cook for 20 minutes, flip halfway through after 10 minutes for medium rare.

6. Remove the steak from the air fryer and place the broccoli florets in the basket.

7. Cook for 5 minutes.

8. Serve the steak with broccoli.

Chipotle Steak

Serving: 2 **Cooking time: 30 minutes**

Nutritional values

Calories 347 kcal

Fat 15.41 g

Total Carbs 4.52 g

Protein 49.01 g

Ingredients

1 lb. beef chuck steak

1 clove garlic, minced

2 red chili, soaked in vinegar for 2 hours

2 tbsp tomato puree

1 1/2 tbsp lemon juice

1/3 tbsp vinegar

1/3 tbsp Worcestershire sauce

1 tsp cumin

Salt to taste

For Garnishing:

2 tbsp parsley, chopped

Some lime, sliced

Directions:

1. In a blender add garlic, chili, tomato puree, lemon juice, vinegar, Worcestershire sauce, cumin and salt; blend until well combined.

2. Place the steaks into a shallow dish and pour the marinade on top. Marinate for 4 hours.

3. Preheat the air fryer to 360F.

4. Place the marinated beef into the air fryer basket and cook for 20 minutes.

5. Once the beef is done, remove from the air fryer and let cool at room temperature.

6. Shred the meat with the help of two forks and return it back to the air fryer.

7.

Lemon Beef Sirloin Roast

Serving: 2   **Cooking time: 50 minutes**

Nutritional values

Calories 376 kcal   Total Carbs 2.96 g

Fat 16.98 g   Protein 53.71 g

Ingredients

1 lbs. beef sirloin roast, boneless

1 1/2 cups beef broth

1 ½ tbsp butter

1/3 tbsp onion powder

1 tsp garlic powder

1 tbsp lemon juice

1/2 tbsp thyme

1/2 tbsp basil

1/2 tbsp oregano

1/2 tbsp rosemary

1/2 tsp dried dill

1/2 tsp black pepper

Salt to taste

Directions:

1. Place the beef in a shallow dish, allowing to come at room temperature.

2. Make a rub by combining lemon juice, onion powder, garlic powder, thyme, basil, oregano, rosemary, dill, black pepper and salt.

3. Rub the mixture all over the beef until evenly coated.

4. Pour the broth, cover and let marinate for at least 6 hours.

5. Grease the air fryer basket with butter and preheat at 400F for 10 minutes.

6. Place the marinated beef into the basket and cook for 30 minutes, flip the roast and continue cooking for another 20 minutes until fall-apart tender.

7. Chop into quarters and serve.

Steak Guacamole Fajitas

Serving: 2   **Cooking time: 25 minutes**

Nutritional values

Calories 231 kcal   Total Carbs 3.41 g

Fat 13.74 g   Protein 23.64 g

Ingredients

2 lbs. trimmed skirt steak, cut into 6 inch crosswise pieces

For Marinade:
1/2 clove garlic, minced
1/2 tbsp Worcestershire sauce
1/2 tbsp taco seasoning
2 tsp ground cumin seeds
1 tsp chili powder
1 tbsp olive oil
1 tsp brown sugar
1/2 tsp ground black pepper
Salt to taste

For Guacamole:
1 small avocado

2 tbsp chopped onion
2 tbsp tomatoes, chopped
1/4 garlic, minced
1 tsp lime juice
1 tbsp cilantro, chopped

For Fajitas:
1/4 cup mozzarella cheese, shredded
1 tbsp sour cream
1/2 small red bell pepper, sliced
1/2 small yellow bell pepper, sliced
1/2 small green bell pepper, sliced
1/4 white onion, sliced
2 tortillas

Directions:

For Guacamole:

1. In a medium mixing bowl, mash avocado, garlic and lime juice.

2. Add in chopped onion, tomatoes and cilantro; mix until well combined.

For Fajitas:

3. Mix all the marinade ingredients to a small mixing bowl.

4. Place the beef in a Ziploc bag and pour the marinade.

5. Marinate for 2 hours.

6. Preheat the air fryer to 360F and grease basket with some oil.

7. Add the marinated beef and sliced peppers to the air fryer and cook at 400F for 20 minutes.

8. Once the beef is cooked through, transfer into a large serving bowl.

9. Spoon about 3 tbsp of the mixture down the center of each tortilla.

10. Add sliced onion and a tbspful of guacamole.

11. Top with some shredded cheese and sour cream; roll up tightly.

12. Place the rolled tortillas, seam side down in the greased air fryer basket and cook for 5 minutes.

13. Serve the wrap warm.

Rosemary Roasted Lamb Leg

Serving: 2　　　**Cooking time: 30 minutes**

Nutritional values

Calories 338 kcal

Fat 11.42 g

Total Carbs 21.4 g

Protein 38.42 g

Ingredients

1 lbs. lamb leg

1 ½ potatoes cut into chunks

1/2 cup peas

1 1/2 clove garlic, minced

1 1/2 tsp oregano

1/2 tsp rosemary

1/2 tsp black pepper

1/2 tbsp olive oil

Salt to taste

For Garnishing:

2 lemon slices

1 tbsp parsley, chopped

Directions:

1. Preheat air fryer to 400F.

2. With the help of sharp knife mark slits in the lamb.

3. Rub the lamb leg with garlic, oregano, rosemary, black pepper, oil and salt.

4. Line the air fryer basket with foil.

5. Place the lamb, potatoes and peas in the basket and cook for 30 minutes.

6. Garnish with parsley and lemon slices.

Citrusy Thyme Chops

Serving: 2　　　**Cooking time: 10 minutes**

Nutritional values

Calories 124 kcal

Fat 5.84 g

Total Carbs 1.31 g

Protein 16.88 g

Ingredients

4 lamb chops

2 tbsp lemon juice

1 tsp rosemary

1 tsp oregano

1 tsp thyme

Salt to taste

Directions:

1. Preheat air fryer to 400F.

2. Season the chops with rosemary, oregano, thyme and salt.

3. Pour in the lemon juice and let marinate for 20 minutes.

4. Place the marinated chops in the air fryer and roast for 10 minutes until nicely brown. Serve warm.

Sweet Potato Steak Delight

Serving: 2 **Cooking time: 12 minutes**

Nutritional values

Calories 343 kcal

Fat 11.5 g

Total Carbs 10.58 g

Protein 49.19 g

Ingredients

1 1/2 lbs. lamb leg steaks-bone-in

1 large sweet potato, cubed

2 tbsp red/white wine vinegar

1 tbsp soy sauce

1/2 tbsp hoisin sauce

1/2 tbsp mustard

1/2 tsp olive oil

Salt and pepper to taste

For Sauce:

1/2 cup tomato sauce

1/2 tbsp soy sauce

1/2 tbsp Worcestershire sauce

1/2 tsp brown sugar

Directions:

For Sauce:

1. Mix all the ingredients to a bowl and microwave for 5 minutes until thick; set aside.

For Lamb:

2. Rub the lamb steaks with little olive oil.

3. Mix vinegar, soy sauce, hoisin sauce, mustard paste, salt and pepper to a mixing bowl.

4. Coat the steaks with the prepared mixture; marinate for 30 minutes.

5. Preheat the air fryer to 360F.

6. Grease the air fryer basket with some oil.

7. Place the steaks and sweet potatoes in the basket and cook for 12 minutes, flip after 6 minutes to evenly brown.

8. Once browned, transfer the steaks and potatoes to a serving dish.

9. Drizzle with sauce and serve.

Spicy Coconut Stir Fry Back Strap

Serving: 2 **Cooking time: 15 minutes**

Nutritional values

Calories 471 kcal

Fat 40.04 g

Total Carbs 6.5 g

Protein 21.63 g

Ingredients

2/3 lbs. lamb fillet or back strap, cut into strips

1/3 cup red bell pepper, cut into strips

1/3 cup mushrooms, sliced

1/3 cup cashews

1 ½ tbsp coconut milk

1/3 tbsp fish sauce

1/3 tbsp curry paste

1/3 tsp brown sugar

1/3 tbsp peanut oil

For Garnishing:

1 tbsp cilantro, chopped

Directions:

1. Combine lamb strips, coconut milk, fish sauce, curry paste, brown sugar and oil to a mixing bowl; cover and place in the refrigerator for 2 hours.

2. Preheat the air fryer to 400F.

3. Place the marinated lamb, veggies and cashews into the basket.

4. Cook for 15 minutes.

5. Garnish with cilantro and serve.

Spring Onion Paprika Dip

Serving: 2   **Cooking time: 15 minutes**

Nutritional values

Calories 45 kcal

Fat 2.01 g

Total Carbs 5.06 g

Protein 2.09 g

Ingredients

1 small onion, preferably Vidalia onion
1/3 cup bread crumbs
1 tsp onion powder
1 tsp garlic powder
2 tsp paprika
1/2 tsp dried thyme
1/2 tsp dried oregano
For Batter:
1/4 cup milk
1 large egg

1 tbsp corn flour
1 tsp oil
1 tsp salt
For Spicy Dip:
1/3 cup mayonnaise
2 sp tomato sauce
1/2 tsp onion powder
1/2 tsp paprika
1/3 tsp sugar
Pinch of chili flakes

Directions:

For Dip:
1. Mix all the ingredients together and set aside.

For Onion:
2. Wash the onion thoroughly and trim the one end off.
3. Set it on flat surface and start cutting downwards to form into a blossom shape.
4. Soak the onion in ice water for at least an hour or overnight to separate the petals.
5. In a mixing bowl, combine bread crumbs, onion powder, garlic powder, paprika, thyme, oregano and salt.
6. In another separate bowl, whisk together eggs, milk and corn flour together.
7. Carefully place the onion into the egg batter. Spoon on top if necessary.
8. Remove from the batter, letting excess drip off.
9. Immediately transfer the onion into the bread crumb mixture, using your hands pat the bread crumbs onto each side of the onion until they are fully covered.
10. Add oil to the bottom of the air fryer and preheat to 400F.
11. Place the onion into the air fryer basket and cook for 15 minutes or until golden and crispy.
12. Once done, carefully remove from the air fryer & serve with the dip.

Cheesypeños

Serving: 2   **Cooking time: 10 minutes**

Nutritional values

Calories 221 kcal

Fat 7.18 g

Total Carbs 28.73 g

Protein 10.17 g

Ingredients

2 large jalapeño peppers

1/3 cup cheddar cheese, shredded

1/3 cup all-purpose flour

2/3 cup bread crumbs

1 egg

1 tsp taco seasoning

Salt to taste

Directions:

1. Cut jalapeno in half lengthwise and remove seeds.
2. In a large mixing bowl, mix flour and eggs together, mix until smooth and lump free; set aside.
3. In another mixing bowl, combine cheddar cheese, taco seasoning and salt.
4. Place the bread crumbs in a shallow bowl.
5. Now spoon 2 tspful of cheese mixture into each jalapeño.
6. Dip each stuffed peppers into the egg batter and then into the bread crumbs.
7. Preheat air fryer to 400F.
8. Add the jalapenos to the preheated air fryer basket, and cook for 10 minutes until browned and crispy.

Vegeterian Corn Burrito

Serving: 2　　**Cooking time: 10 minutes**

Nutritional values

Calories 312 kcal

Fat 12.05 g

Total Carbs 48.77 g

Protein 11.43 g

Ingredients

8 corn tortillas

2 large egg plant, sliced

1 cup broccoli florets

1-1/4 cups, tin black beans, drained

1 large avocado, sliced

1 cup sweet corn

1 small head lettuce, chopped

1/4 cup cilantro, chopped

1 clove garlic, minced

1 tsp cumin

1 tsp chili powder

1 tsp paprika

1/2 tsp salt

For Salsa:

1 cup tomatoes, chopped

1 cup cucumber, chopped

1 tbsp lemon juice

Salt and black pepper to taste

For Garnishing:

Sour cream

Fresh parsley

Directions:

1. Season the eggplant and broccoli with garlic, cumin, chili powder, paprika and salt.
2. Preheat the air fryer to 400F.
3. Place the seasoned eggplant and broccoli in the air fryer.
4. Cook for about 10 minutes.

For Salsa:

5. In a small mixing bowl, combine all the salsa ingredients and set aside.

Assembling:

6. To assemble the vegan burrito bowl, place eggplant and broccoli into the bottom of the bowl.
7. Layer with black bean mixture.
8. Add avocado, sweet corn and cilantro.
9. Top with a spoonful of salsa and a dollop of sour cream.
10. Decorate the edges with the tortilla chips.
11. Top with shredded lettuce and parsley.

Aubergine Pizza

Serving: 2　　**Cooking time: 15 minutes**

Nutritional values

Calories 201 kcal

Fat 8.26 g

Total Carbs 18.04 g

Protein 14.8 g

Ingredients

1lbs. eggplant

1/2 cup pizza sauce

1/2 cup breadcrumbs

1/2 cup mozzarella cheese

1/2 cup cheddar cheese

1 small egg

1/2 tbsp taco seasoning

Directions:

1. Preheat the air fryer to 360F.
2. Cut eggplant into 1-inch thick disc.
3. In a mixing bowl, whisk egg until frothy.
4. In a medium shallow plate, combine breadcrumbs and taco seasoning.
5. Dip each eggplant slice into the egg and then into the breadcrumb mixture to coat evenly.
6. Now place a spoonful of pizza sauce.
7. Top with cheese.
8. Place the prepared eggplant in the air fryer basket.
9. Cook for 15 minutes until cheese is melted.

Butter Cocoa Brownies

Serving: 2   **Cooking time: 20 minutes**

Nutritional values

Calories 363 kcal

Fat 23.87 g

Total Carbs 35.86 g

Protein 4.45 g

Ingredients

1/3 cup flour

1/3 cup sugar

6 tbsp butter

1 ½ tbsp cocoa powder

1/2 tsp baking powder

1 egg

1/2 tsp vanilla extract

1 pinch of salt

For Serving:

Vanilla ice cream

Directions:

1. Preheat the air fryer to 350F and grease a baking tin with non-stick spray.

2. In a mixing bowl, sift together flour, cocoa powder, baking powder and salt; set aside.

3. In another mixing bowl, beat butter, sugar and vanilla extract together, beat until light and fluffy.

4. Add eggs and whisk again until pale and creamy.

5. Now fold in the dry ingredients and mix until well combined.

6. Pour the batter into the prepared pan.

7. Set the pan in the air fryer basket and bake for 20 minutes or until toothpick inserted out comes clean.

8. Top with vanilla ice cream and serve.

Tropical Cookies

Serving: 2   **Cooking time: 15 minutes**

Nutritional values

Calories 243 kcal

Fat 13.9 g

Total Carbs 27.64 g

Protein 2.44 g

Ingredients

1/4 cup flour

3 tbsp sugar

3 tbsp coconut, shredded

2 tbsp butter

1/2 tsp baking powder

1/2 tbsp cornstarch

1 small egg

1/2 tsp coconut or vanilla extract

Directions:

1. In a mixing bowl, beat butter & sugar until light & fluffy.

2. Add eggs and coconut extract, beat again.

3. In another mixing bowl, combine flour, cornstarch and baking powder together.

4. Add dry ingredients and continue beating until mixture turns into a dough.

5. Fold in the shredded coconut.

6. Wrap the dough into a plastic wrap and refrigerate for at least 2 hours.

7. Form 1-inch balls and place on to a large serving plate.

8. Slightly flatten the balls with the back of the spoon.

9. Line the air fryer basket with parchment paper and preheat the air fryer to 360F.

10. Carefully place the cookies in the basket with a little gap in between each other.

11. Cook for about 15 minutes until slightly golden brown.

Chocolate Chip Cake

Serving: 2　　**Cooking time: 15 minutes**

Nutritional values

Calories 350 kcal

Fat 24.31 g

Total Carbs 27.31 g

Protein 6.7 g

Ingredients

6 tbsp chocolate chips

2 tbsp butter

2 small eggs, separated

2 tbsp sugar

1 tbsp cocoa powder

1/2 tsp vanilla extract

1 tbsp powdered sugar, for dusting

Directions:

1. Preheat air fryer to 400F and lightly butter 4 ramekin dishes.

2. Melt chocolate chips and butter together, either in the microwave or in a double boiler.

3. Remove from heat and let cool to room temperature, about 10 minutes.

4. Stir in the egg yolks, sugar, cocoa powder and vanilla extract; mix until well combined.

5. In a separated large bowl, using an electric mixer beat egg whites until soft peaks are formed.

6. Fold the whites into the yolk mixture.

7. Transfer the batter carefully to the buttered ramekins, taking care not to get on top edge of the ramekins.

8. Now carefully place the ramekins in the air fryer and bake for 15 minutes until puffed.

9. Dust with powdered sugar and serve immediately.

Instant Pot Choco Doughnuts

Serving: 2　　**Cooking time: 10 minutes**

Nutritional values

Calories 196 kcal

Fat 7.84 g

Total Carbs 27.62 g

Protein 3.62 g

Ingredients

For Donuts:
1/2 cups all-purpose flour
1 1/2 tbsp butter, cold cut into cubes
1 ½ tbsp milk
1 tbsp sugar
1/2 tsp baking powder
For Topping:
1/4 cup melted Chocolate

For Glaze:
1/4 cup powdered sugar
Pink food coloring
1 drop vanilla extract
2 tsp water
For Cinnamon Sugar:
2 tbsp powdered sugar
1 pinch of cinnamon

Directions:

For Glaze:
1. Mix powdered sugar, food color, vanilla extract and water to a bowl; mix until thick paste consistency.
For Cinnamon Sugar:
2. Mix cinnamon and sugar together in a bowl & set aside.
For Donuts:
3. In a large mixing bowl, combine flour, sugar and baking powder.
4. Add the cubed butter, using your fingers crumble the mixture.
5. Add milk and knead until dough comes together.
6. Transfer the mixture onto a lightly floured surface and knead until dough is no more-sticky.
7. Wrap the dough in a plastic wrap and refrigerate for at least 30 minutes to set.
8. Roll the dough into a 1/8 inch-thick rectangle.
9. Using a donut cutter cut circles out of the dough.
10. Preheat air fryer to 400F and lightly butter the air fryer basket with some oil.
11. Place the 4 donuts in the air fryer at a time, spacing evenly to avoid touching.
12. Cook for 10 minutes until browned and puffed.
13. Once the donuts are browned, immediately roll some donuts into the cinnamon sugar mixture.
14. Dip some into the glaze and chocolate sauce.
15. Place on a wire rack to cool.
16. Serve and enjoy.

MONTHLY SCHEDULES

I hope you enjoyed the book so far and are already
cooking the delicious recipes included.

Get started and cook all the recipes included in
this book!

WEEK 1	Monday	Tuesday	Wednesday	Thursday	Friday	saturday	sunday
Meal 1	Chicken Wings	Turkey Burgers	Chicken Sandwich	Beef chipotle	Chocolate Soufflé	Eggplant Pizza	Teriyaki Beef Steak with Broccoli
Meal 2	Herb Crusted Pork Ribs	Vegan Tacos	BBQ Pulled Pork with Coleslaw	Chocolate Fudge Brownies	Crispy Coconut Pork Belly	Lamb Pie	Sticky Lemon Drumsticks
Meal3	Blooming Onion with Spicy dip	Beef Kabobs	Coconut Cookies	Spicy Lamb Meatballs with Mango Salsa	Butter-Honey Glazed Turkey	Pineapple Turkey Kabobs	Roasted Lamb Leg

WEEK 2	Monday	Tuesday	Wednesday	Thursday	Friday	saturday	sunday
Meal 1	Vegan Burrito Bowl	Turkey Pattie with Avocado Salad	Pork Quesadillas	Kale chips	Lamb Steak with Sweet Potatoes	Cheesy Jalapenos	Thai Lamb Stir Fry
Meal 2	Rotisserie Chicken	Assorted Donuts	Crispy Garlic Chicken with Lemon Dip	Cinnamon Sugar Churros	Pork Steaks with Broccoli	Pistachio Stuffed Turkey Breast	Pineapple Bites
Meal3	Pork Dumplings	Skirt Steak Fajitas Wraps	Sweet and Sour Lamb Ribs	Beef Stuffed Capsicum	Mexican Turkey Tacos	Spaghetti Meatballs on Stick	Tandoori Masala Chicken

WEEK 3	Monday	Tuesday	Wednesday	Thursday	Friday	saturday	sunday
Meal 1	Chicken Nuggets	Turkey Quesadilla	Vegetable Fritters	Veggie Stuffed Peppers	Chicken Pie	Vegetable Lasagna	Chinese beef and Broccoli
Meal 2	Lemon Herb Lamb Chops	Chocolate Cake	Balsamic Pork	BBQ Pork Sandwich	Cheesy Zucchini boat	Beef and Mushroom Meatloaf	Sweet and Sour Cauliflower Stir fry
Meal3	Crispy Mongolian Beef	Classic Lamb Shanks	Apricot Glazed Turkey Legs	Roasted Almond Chicken	Basil Lamb Cutlets	Lemon Garlic Turkey	Buttery Pork Chops

WEEK 4	Monday	Tuesday	Wednesday	Thursday	Friday	saturday	sunday
Meal 1	Mexican Chicken Wrap	Potato Croquettes	Black Bean Burger	Tropical Egg Rolls	Sweet Potato Jackets	Raisin Bread Pudding with Chocolate	Vegetable Spring rolls
Meal 2	Pork Medallions with Sour Cream	Pulled Turkey Sandwich	Crispy Pork	Mediterranean Lamb Burgers	Lemon Pork Ribs	Cranberry Turkey Wings	Almond Stuffed Chicken
Meal3	Turkish Kebabs with Tahini Sauce	Thai Beef Salad	Lemon Herb Beef Roast	Turkey Meatloaf	Crispy Cheesy Lamb Chops	Thai Chicken Skewers	Salted beef with Caramelized Onions

WEEK 5	Monday	Tuesday	Wednesday	Thursday	Friday	saturday	sunday
Meal 1	Chicken Lollipops	Buffalo Cauliflower Wings	Blueberry Cheesecake	Vegetable Sushi	Tofu Satay	Sticky BBQ Tofu	Classic Falafel
Meal 2	Beef with Mix Vegetables	Turkey Sausages	Honey Mustard Pork Chops	Chicken Wings	Cheese Stuffed Turkey Meatballs	Sticky BBQ Honey Strips	BBQ Chicken Pizza
Meal3	Plum Roast Lamb	BBQ Pulled Pork with Coleslaw	Walnut-Stuffed Lamb	Beef chipotle	Spicy Lamb Meatballs with Mango Salsa	Pork Shoulder Skewers with Pineapple	Butter-Honey Glazed Turkey

WEEK 6	Monday	Tuesday	Wednesday	Thursday	Friday	saturday	sunday
Meal 1	Chicken Sandwich	Cheesy Jalapenos	Pork Dumplings	Tandoori Masala Chicken	Pork Quesadillas	Lamb Pie	Chocolate Fudge Brownies
Meal 2	Skirt Steak Fajitas Wraps	Mexican Turkey Tacos	Blooming Onion with Spicy dip	Teriyaki Beef Steak with Broccoli	Pineapple Bites	Kale chips	Herb Crusted Pork Ribs
Meal 3	Pistachio Stuffed Turkey Breast	Beef Kabobs	Roasted Lamb Leg	Assorted Donuts	Lamb Steak with Sweet Potatoes	Crispy Garlic Chicken with Lemon Dip	Pineapple Turkey Kabobs

WEEK 7	Monday	Tuesday	Wednesday	Thursday	Friday	saturday	sunday
Meal 1	Sticky Lemon Drumsticks	Eggplant Pizza	Turkey Burgers	Chocolate Soufflé	Vegan Burrito Bowl	Turkey Pattie with Avocado Salad	Vegan Tacos
Meal 2	Cinnamon Sugar Churros	Pork Steaks with Broccoli	Coconut Cookies	Spaghetti Meatballs on Stick	Sweet and Sour Lamb Ribs	Roasted Almond Chicken	Thai Lamb Stir Fry
Meal 3	Crispy Coconut Pork Belly	Apricot Glazed Turkey Legs	Buttery Pork Chops	Chinese beef and Broccoli	Classic Lamb Shanks	Beef Stuffed Capsicum	Rotisserie Chicken

WEEK 8	Monday	Tuesday	Wednesday	Thursday	Friday	saturday	sunday
Meal 1	Chicken Nuggets	Veggie Stuffed Peppers	Chicken Pie	Sweet and Sour Cauliflower Stir fry	Cheesy Zucchini boat	Mexican Chicken Wrap	Raisin Bread Pudding with Chocolate
Meal 2	Crispy Pork	Cranberry Turkey Wings	Potato Croquettes	Pulled Turkey Sandwich	Basil Lamb Cutlets	Vegetable Fritters	Lemon Garlic Turkey
Meal 3	Beef and Mushroom Meatloaf	Mediterranean Lamb Burgers	Lemon Herb Beef Roast	Lemon Herb Lamb Chops	Crispy Mongolian Beef	Lemon Pork Ribs	Balsamic Pork

WEEK 9	Monday	Tuesday	Wednesday	Thursday	Friday	saturday	sunday
Meal 1	Vegetable Lasagna	Turkey Quesadilla	Sweet Potato Jackets	BBQ Pork Sandwich	Black Bean Burger	Tropical Egg Rolls	Vegetable Spring rolls
Meal 2	Almond Stuffed Chicken	Chocolate Cake	Pork Medallions with Sour Cream	Thai Beef Salad	Crispy Cheesy Lamb Chops	Beef with Mix Vegetables	Turkey Meatloaf
Meal 3	Honey Mustard Pork Chops	Turkish Kebabs with Tahini Sauce	Chicken Lollipops	Butter-Honey Glazed Turkey	Thai Chicken Skewers	Plum Roast Lamb	Salted beef with Caramelized Onions

WEEK 10	Monday	Tuesday	Wednesday	Thursday	Friday	saturday	sunday
Meal 1	BBQ Chicken Pizza	Buffalo Cauliflower Wings	Classic Falafel	Cheese Stuffed Turkey Meatballs	Vegetable Sushi	Chicken Wings	Blooming Onion with Spicy dip
Meal 2	Pork Dumplings	Pineapple Turkey Kabobs	Pork Shoulder Skewers with Pineapple	Chocolate Fudge Brownies	Tandoori Masala Chicken	Blueberry Cheesecake	Spicy Lamb Meatballs with Mango Salsa
Meal 3	Walnut-Stuffed Lamb	Beef chipotle	BBQ Pulled Pork with Coleslaw	Teriyaki Beef Steak with Broccoli	Roasted Lamb Leg	Mexican Turkey Tacos	Sticky BBQ Honey Strips

11	Monday	Tuesday	Wednesday	Thursday	Friday	saturday	sunday
Meal 1	Tofu Satay	Chicken Sandwich	Assorted Donuts	Turkey Sausages	Cheesy Jalapenos	Pork Quesadillas	Skirt Steak Fajitas Wraps
Meal 2	Crispy Garlic Chicken with Lemon Dip	Pistachio Stuffed Turkey Breast	Pineapple Bites	Sticky Lemon Drumsticks	Turkey Pattie with Avocado Salad	Coconut Cookies	Lamb Pie
Meal3	Spaghetti Meatballs on Stick	Lamb Steak with Sweet Potatoes	Pork Steaks with Broccoli	Kale chips	Sweet and Sour Lamb Ribs	Herb Crusted Pork Ribs	Beef Kabobs

WEEK 12	Monday	Tuesday	Wednesday	Thursday	Friday	saturday	sunday
Meal 1	Eggplant Pizza	Chicken Nuggets	Sticky BBQ Tofu	Turkey Burgers	Cheesy Zucchini boat	Rotisserie Chicken	Chocolate Soufflé
Meal 2	Cinnamon Sugar Churros	Crispy Coconut Pork Belly	Classic Lamb Shanks	Vegan Tacos	Buttery Pork Chops	Beef Stuffed Capsicum	Basil Lamb Cutlets
Meal3	Roasted Almond Chicken	Lemon Garlic Turkey	Balsamic Pork	Crispy Mongolian Beef	Apricot Glazed Turkey Legs	Thai Lamb Stir Fry	Chinese beef and Broccoli

WEEK 13	Monday	Tuesday	Wednesday	Thursday	Friday	saturday	sunday
Meal 1	Veggie Stuffed Peppers	Potato Croquettes	Vegetable Spring rolls	Sweet and Sour Cauliflower Stir fry	Vegetable Fritters	Black Bean Burger	Mexican Chicken Wrap
Meal 2	Chicken Pie	Pulled Turkey Sandwich	BBQ Pork Sandwich	Mediterranean Lamb Burgers	Beef and Mushroom Meatloaf	Almond Stuffed Chicken	Turkey Meatloaf
Meal3	Cranberry Turkey Wings	Crispy Pork	Lemon Herb Beef Roast	Salted beef with Caramelized Onions	Turkish Kebabs with Tahini Sauce	Lemon Pork Ribs	Lemon Herb Lamb Chops

WEEK 14	Monday	Tuesday	Wednesday	Thursday	Friday	saturday	sunday
Meal 1	Thai Chicken Skewers	Turkey Quesadilla	Pork Dumplings	Sweet Potato Jackets	Vegan Burrito Bowl	Vegetable Lasagna	Raisin Bread Pudding with Chocolate
Meal 2	Chicken Lollipops	Chocolate Cake	Honey Mustard Pork Chops	Beef with Mix Vegetables	Plum Roast Lamb	BBQ Chicken Pizza	Cheese Stuffed Turkey Meatballs
Meal3	Butter-Honey Glazed Turkey	Walnut-Stuffed Lamb	Thai Beef Salad	Sticky BBQ Honey Strips	Pork Medallions with Sour Cream	Crispy Cheesy Lamb Chops	Tropical Egg Rolls

WEEK 15	Monday	Tuesday	Wednesday	Thursday	Friday	saturday	sunday
Meal 1	Chicken Wings	Buffalo Cauliflower Wings	Teriyaki Beef Steak with Broccoli	Spicy Lamb Meatballs with Mango Salsa	Vegetable Sushi	Cheesy Jalapenos	Lamb Steak with Sweet Potatoes
Meal 2	Blueberry Cheesecake	Mexican Turkey Tacos	Classic Falafel	Coconut Cookies	Roasted Lamb Leg	Pork Shoulder Skewers with Pineapple	Beef chipotle
Meal3	Herb Crusted Pork Ribs	Crispy Garlic Chicken with Lemon Dip	BBQ Pulled Pork with Coleslaw	Pineapple Turkey Kabobs	Pistachio Stuffed Turkey Breast	Beef Kabobs	Tandoori Masala Chi

WEEK 16	Monday	Tuesday	Wednesday	Thursday	Friday	saturday	sunday
Meal 1	Blooming Onion with Spicy dip	Turkey Sausages	Pork Quesadillas	Skirt Steak Fajitas Wraps	Chicken Sandwich	Lamb Pie	Turkey Burgers
Meal 2	Kale chips	Tofu Satay	Chocolate Fudge Brownies	Pineapple Bites	Sweet and Sour Lamb Ribs	Sticky Lemon Drumsticks	Assorted Donuts
Meal 3	Roasted Almond Chicken	Classic Lamb Shanks	Turkey Pattie with Avocado Salad	Chinese beef and Broccoli	Pork Steaks with Broccoli	Crispy Coconut Pork Belly	Spaghetti Meatballs on Stick

WEEK 17	Monday	Tuesday	Wednesday	Thursday	Friday	saturday	sunday
Meal 1	Rotisserie Chicken	Vegan Tacos	Thai Lamb Stir Fry	Eggplant Pizza	Chicken Nuggets	Cheesy Zucchini boat	Sticky BBQ Tofu
Meal 2	Chicken Pie	Crispy Pork	Balsamic Pork	Chocolate Soufflé	Basil Lamb Cutlets	Cinnamon Sugar Churros	Buttery Pork Chops
Meal 3	Lemon Garlic Turkey	Lemon Herb Lamb Chops	Cranberry Turkey Wings	Beef and Mushroom Meatloaf	Beef Stuffed Capsicum	Crispy Mongolian Beef	Apricot Glazed Turkey Legs

WEEK 18	Monday	Tuesday	Wednesday	Thursday	Friday	saturday	sunday
Meal 1	Mexican Chicken Wrap	Veggie Stuffed Peppers	Turkey Meatloaf	Thai Chicken Skewers	Pulled Turkey Sandwich	Potato Croquettes	Sweet and Sour Cauliflower Stir fry
Meal 2	Vegetable Spring rolls	Mediterranean Lamb Burgers	BBQ Pork Sandwich	Salted beef with Caramelized Onions	Vegetable Fritters	Almond Stuffed Chicken	Black Bean Burger
Meal 3	Plum Roast Lamb	Butter-Honey Glazed Turkey	Lemon Herb Beef Roast	Sticky BBQ Honey Strips	Turkish Kebabs with Tahini Sauce	Lemon Pork Ribs	Pork Dumplings

WEEK 19	Monday	Tuesday	Wednesday	Thursday	Friday	saturday	sunday
Meal 1	Chicken Lollipops	Turkey Quesadilla	BBQ Chicken Pizza	Vegan Burrito Bowl	Vegetable Lasagna	Sweet Potato Jackets	Raisin Bread Pudding with Chocolate
Meal 2	Chocolate Cake	Cheese Stuffed Turkey Meatballs	Chicken Wings	Tropical Egg Rolls	Walnut-Stuffed Lamb	Beef with Mix Vegetables	Thai Beef Salad
Meal 3	Spicy Lamb Meatballs with Mango Salsa	Beef chipotle	Pork Medallions with Sour Cream	Honey Mustard Pork Chops	Pork Shoulder Skewers with Pineapple	Pineapple Turkey Kabobs	Crispy Cheesy Lamb Chops

WEEK 20	Monday	Tuesday	Wednesday	Thursday	Friday	saturday	sunday
Meal 1	Tandoori Masala Chicken	Mexican Turkey Tacos	Vegetable Sushi	Cheesy Jalapenos	Buffalo Cauliflower Wings	Sticky Lemon Drumsticks	Blueberry Cheesecake
Meal 2	Teriyaki Beef Steak with Broccoli	Coconut Cookies	Crispy Garlic Chicken with Lemon Dip	BBQ Pulled Pork with Coleslaw	Lamb Steak with Sweet Potatoes	Pork Steaks with Broccoli	Classic Falafel
Meal 3	Turkey Pattie h Avocado lad	Herb Crusted Pork Ribs	Roasted Lamb Leg	Skirt Steak Fajitas Wraps	Pistachio Stuffed Turkey Breast	Beef Kabobs	Sweet and Sour Lamb Ribs

21	Monday	Tuesday	Wednesday	Thursday	Friday	saturday	sunday
Meal 1	Chicken Sandwich	Turkey Sausages	Blooming Onion with Spicy dip	Spaghetti Meatballs on Stick	Lamb Pie	Tofu Satay	Pork Quesadillas
Meal 2	Kale chips	Pineapple Bites	Beef Stuffed Capsicum	Buttery Pork Chops	Assorted Donuts	Thai Lamb Stir Fry	Chocolate Fudge Brownies
Meal 3	Crispy Coconut Pork Belly	Rotisserie Chicken	Roasted Almond Chicken	Chinese beef and Broccoli	Apricot Glazed Turkey Legs	Classic Lamb Shanks	Turkey Burgers

WEEK 22	Monday	Tuesday	Wednesday	Thursday	Friday	saturday	sunday
Meal 1	Sticky BBQ Tofu	Mexican Chicken Wrap	Eggplant Pizza	Chicken Pie	Cheesy Zucchini boat	Pulled Turkey Sandwich	Chicken Nuggets
Meal 2	Crispy Pork	Vegan Tacos	Beef and Mushroom Meatloaf	Cinnamon Sugar Churros	Cranberry Turkey Wings	Crispy Mongolian Beef	Chocolate Soufflé
Meal 3	Lemon Herb Beef Roast	Lemon Garlic Turkey	Lemon Herb Lamb Chops	Lemon Pork Ribs	Turkish Kebabs with Tahini Sauce	Balsamic Pork	Basil Lamb Cutlets

WEEK 23	Monday	Tuesday	Wednesday	Thursday	Friday	saturday	sunday
Meal 1	Veggie Stuffed Peppers	Chicken Lollipops	Potato Croquettes	Sweet and Sour Cauliflower Stir fry	Vegetable Fritters	Turkey Quesadilla	Black Bean Burger
Meal 2	Pork Dumplings	Vegetable Spring rolls	Turkey Meatloaf	Sticky BBQ Honey Strips	BBQ Pork Sandwich	Mediterranean Lamb Burgers	Crispy Cheesy Lamb Chops
Meal 3	Thai Chicken Skewers	Butter-Honey Glazed Turkey	Pork Medallions with Sour Cream	Plum Roast Lamb	Salted beef with Caramelized Onions	Almond Stuffed Chicken	Thai Beef Salad

WEEK 24	Monday	Tuesday	Wednesday	Thursday	Friday	saturday	sunday
Meal 1	Chicken Wings	Sweet Potato Jackets	Chocolate Cake	Vegan Burrito Bowl	Raisin Bread Pudding with Chocolate	Beef with Mix Vegetables	Tropical Egg Rolls
Meal 2	Beef chipotle	Spicy Lamb Meatballs with Mango Salsa	Crispy Garlic Chicken with Lemon Dip	Lamb Steak with Sweet Potatoes	BBQ Chicken Pizza	Vegetable Lasagna	Honey Mustard Pork Chops
Meal 3	Pork Shoulder Skewers with Pineapple	Pistachio Stuffed Turkey Breast	Teriyaki Beef Steak with Broccoli	Cheese Stuffed Turkey Meatballs	BBQ Pulled Pork with Coleslaw	Pineapple Turkey Kabobs	Walnut-Stuffed Lamb

WEEK 25	Monday	Tuesday	Wednesday	Thursday	Friday	saturday	sunday
Meal 1	Pork Steaks with Broccoli	Buffalo Cauliflower Wings	Sticky Lemon Drumsticks	Vegetable Sushi	Cheesy Jalapenos	Coconut Cookies	Blueberry Cheesecake
Meal 2	Classic Falafel	Turkey Pattie with Avocado Salad	Skirt Steak Fajitas Wraps	Sweet and Sour Lamb Ribs	Chicken Sandwich	Lamb Pie	Mexican Turk Tacos
Meal 3	Beef Kabobs	Roasted Lamb Leg	Pork Quesadillas	Turkey Sausages	Herb Crusted Pork Ribs	Spaghetti Meatballs on Stick	Tand Masala

88

WEEK 26	Monday	Tuesday	Wednesday	Thursday	Friday	saturday	sunday
Meal 1	Blooming Onion with Spicy dip	Turkey Burgers	Tofu Satay	Rotisserie Chicken	Kale chips	Chinese beef and Broccoli	Thai Lamb Stir Fry
Meal 2	Crispy Coconut Pork Belly	Mexican Chicken Wrap	Buttery Pork Chops	Assorted Donuts	Lemon Pork Ribs	Chocolate Fudge Brownies	Pineapple Bites
Meal 3	Lemon Herb Lamb Chops	Beef Stuffed Capsicum	Classic Lamb Shanks	Cranberry Turkey Wings	Roasted Almond Chicken	Apricot Glazed Turkey Legs	Crispy Mongolian Beef

WEEK 27	Monday	Tuesday	Wednesday	Thursday	Friday	saturday	sunday
Meal 1	Sweet and Sour Cauliflower Stir fry	Chicken Nuggets	Potato Croquettes	Vegan Tacos	Basil Lamb Cutlets	Eggplant Pizza	Sticky BBQ Tofu
Meal 2	BBQ Pork Sandwich	Pulled Turkey Sandwich	Chocolate Soufflé	Chicken Pie	Turkey Meatloaf	Salted beef with Caramelized Onions	Mediterranean Lamb Burgers
Meal 3	Lemon Herb Beef Roast	Turkish Kebabs with Tahini Sauce	Crispy Pork	Beef and Mushroom Meatloaf	Balsamic Pork	Almond Stuffed Chicken	Lemon Garlic Turkey

WEEK 28	Monday	Tuesday	Wednesday	Thursday	Friday	saturday	sunday
Meal 1	Black Bean Burger	Turkey Quesadilla	Pork Dumplings	Sweet Potato Jackets	Chicken Lollipops	Vegetable Spring rolls	Tropical Egg Rolls
Meal 2	Chicken Wings	Spicy Lamb Meatballs with Mango Salsa	Chocolate Cake	Crispy Cheesy Lamb Chops	Pork Medallions with Sour Cream	Vegetable Lasagna	Beef with Mix Vegetables
Meal 3	Pork Shoulder Skewers with Pineapple	Sticky BBQ Honey Strips	Thai Chicken Skewers	Butter-Honey Glazed Turkey	Thai Beef Salad	Plum Roast Lamb	Pineapple Turkey Kabobs

WEEK 29	Monday	Tuesday	Wednesday	Thursday	Friday	saturday	sunday
Meal 1	Teriyaki Beef Steak with Broccoli	Raisin Bread Pudding with Chocolate	Crispy Garlic Chicken with Lemon Dip	Beef chipotle	Cheesy Zucchini boat	Mexican Turkey Tacos	Pork Steaks with Broccoli
Meal 2	Roasted Lamb Leg	Pistachio Stuffed Turkey Breast	Walnut-Stuffed Lamb	Cinnamon Sugar Churros	Lamb Steak with Sweet Potatoes	Veggie Stuffed Peppers	Vegetable Fritters
Meal 3	Tandoori Masala Chicken	Vegan Burrito Bowl	Honey Mustard Pork Chops	Cheese Stuffed Turkey Meatballs	BBQ Pulled Pork with Coleslaw	BBQ Chicken Pizza	Beef Kabobs

WEEK 30	Monday	Tuesday	Wednesday	Thursday	Friday	saturday	sunday
Meal 1	Lemon Pork Ribs	Crispy Mongolian Beef	Sweet and Sour Lamb Ribs	Apricot Glazed Turkey Legs	Roasted Almond Chicken	Crispy Coconut Pork Belly	Beef Stuffed Capsicum
Meal 2	Cheesy Jalapenos	Classic Falafel	Blooming Onion with Spicy dip	Pineapple Bites	Vegetable Sushi	Blueberry Cheesecake	Mexican Chicken Wrap
Meal 3	Sausages	Sticky Lemon Drumsticks	Pork Quesadillas	Spaghetti Meatballs on Stick	Lemon Herb Lamb Chops	Turkey Burgers	Classic Lamb Shanks

WEEK 31	Monday	Tuesday	Wednesday	Thursday	Friday	saturday	sunday
Meal 1	Chicken Sandwich	Turkey Pattie with Avocado Salad	Herb Crusted Pork Ribs	Skirt Steak Fajitas Wraps	Roasted Lamb Leg	Chicken Nuggets	Cranberry Turkey Wings
Meal 2	Buffalo Cauliflower Wings	Coconut Cookies	Tofu Satay	Chocolate Fudge Brownies	Kale Chips	Assorted Donuts	Chinese beef and Broccoli
Meal3	Beef and Mushroom Meatloaf	Lamb Pie	Rotisserie Chicken	Buttery Pork Chops	Lemon Garlic Turkey	Balsamic Pork	Thai Lamb Stir Fry

WEEK 32	Monday	Tuesday	Wednesday	Thursday	Friday	saturday	sunday
Meal 1	Chicken Pie	Turkey Meatloaf	Thai Chicken Skewers	Butter-Honey Glazed Turkey	Chicken Lollipops	Turkey Quesadilla	Pork Dumplings
Meal 2	Sticky BBQ Honey Strips	Pork Medallions with Sour Cream	Thai Beef Salad	BBQ Pork Sandwich	Salted beef with Caramelized Onions	Vegetable Spring rolls	Sticky BBQ Tofu
Meal3	Potato Croquettes	Basil Lamb Cutlets	Tropical Egg Rolls	Plum Roast Lamb	Eggplant Pizza	Sweet and Sour Cauliflower Stir fry	Turkish Kebabs with Tahini Sauce

WEEK 33	Monday	Tuesday	Wednesday	Thursday	Friday	saturday	sunday
Meal 1	Beef with Mix Vegetables	Crispy Cheesy Lamb Chops	Beef chipotle	Honey Mustard Pork Chops	Spicy Lamb Meatballs with Mango Salsa	Lemon Herb Beef Roast	Mediterranean Lamb Burgers
Meal 2	Chicken Wings	Pineapple Turkey Kabobs	BBQ Chicken Pizza	Cheese Stuffed Turkey Meatballs	Almond Stuffed Chicken	Pork Shoulder Skewers with Pineapple	Pulled Turkey Sandwich
Meal3	Chocolate Soufflé	Crispy Pork	Vegetable Lasagna	Black Bean Burger	Sweet Potato Jackets	Chocolate Cake	Vegan Tacos

WEEK 34	Monday	Tuesday	Wednesday	Thursday	Friday	saturday	sunday
Meal 1	Sticky Lemon Drumsticks	Mexican Turkey Tacos	Roasted Almond Chicken	Teriyaki Beef Steak with Broccoli	Apricot Glazed Turkey Legs	Crispy Garlic Chicken with Lemon Dip	Turkey Sausages
Meal 2	Lemon Pork Ribs	Walnut-Stuffed Lamb	Pork Quesadillas	Lamb Steak with Sweet Potatoes	Pork Steaks with Broccoli	Sweet and Sour Lamb Ribs	Spaghetti Meatballs on Stick
Meal3	Vegetable Fritters	Veggie Stuffed Peppers	Crispy Mongolian Beef	Cinnamon Sugar Churros	Cheesy Zucchini boat	Blueberry Cheesecake	Vegetable Sushi

WEEK 35	Monday	Tuesday	Wednesday	Thursday	Friday	saturday	sunday
Meal 1	Vegan Burrito Bowl	Mexican Chicken Wrap	Cheesy Jalapenos	Coconut Cookies	Chicken Sandwich	Blooming Onion with Spicy dip	Tandoori Masala Chicken
Meal 2	Classic Falafel	Crispy Coconut Pork Belly	Classic Lamb Shanks	Buttery Pork Chops	Lemon Herb Lamb Chops	BBQ Pulled Pork with Coleslaw	Roasted Lamb Leg
Meal3	Skirt Steak Fajitas Wraps	Turkey Pattie with Avocado Salad	Beef Stuffed Capsicum	Pistachio Stuffed Turkey Breast	Beef Kabobs	Turkey Burgers	Pineapple Bites

WEEK 36	Monday	Tuesday	Wednesday	Thursday	Friday	saturday	sunday
Meal 1	Chocolate Fudge Brownies	Tofu Satay	Sweet and Sour Cauliflower Stir fry	Chicken Nuggets	Eggplant Pizza	Buffalo Cauliflower Wings	Chicken Lollipops
Meal 2	Thai Chicken Skewers	Turkey Meatloaf	BBQ Pork Sandwich	Salted beef with Caramelized Onions	Thai Lamb Stir Fry	Assorted Donuts	Pork Dumplings
Meal 3	Turkish Kebabs with Tahini Sauce	Thai Beef Salad	Roasted Lamb Leg	Balsamic Pork	Lemon Garlic Turkey	Chinese beef and Broccoli	Butter-Honey Glazed Turkey

WEEK 37	Monday	Tuesday	Wednesday	Thursday	Friday	saturday	sunday
Meal 1	Potato Croquettes	Tropical Egg Rolls	Vegetable Spring rolls	Chicken Pie	Chocolate Soufflé	Kale chips	Sticky BBQ Tofu
Meal 2	Lamb Pie	Turkey Quesadilla	Plum Roast Lamb	Pulled Turkey Sandwich	Basil Lamb Cutlets	Crispy Pork	Cranberry Turkey Wings
Meal 3	Almond Stuffed Chicken	Lemon Herb Beef Roast	Herb Crusted Pork Ribs	Sticky BBQ Honey Strips	Rotisserie Chicken	Beef and Mushroom Meatloaf	Pork Medallions with Sour Cream

WEEK 38	Monday	Tuesday	Wednesday	Thursday	Friday	saturday	sunday
Meal 1	Pork Shoulder Skewers with Pineapple	Pineapple Turkey Kabobs	Beef with Mix Vegetables	Pork Steaks with Broccoli	Teriyaki Beef Steak with Broccoli	Lemon Pork Ribs	Crispy Mongolian Beef
Meal 2	Crispy Garlic Chicken with Lemon Dip	Crispy Cheesy Lamb Chops	Roasted Almond Chicken	Walnut-Stuffed Lamb	Vegan Tacos	Turkey Sausages	Mediterranean Lamb Burgers
Meal 3	Cinnamon Sugar Churros	Vegetable Lasagna	Mexican Turkey Tacos	Vegetable Fritters	Chicken Wings	Black Bean Burger	Cheesy Zucchini boat

WEEK 39	Monday	Tuesday	Wednesday	Thursday	Friday	saturday	sunday
Meal 1	BBQ Chicken Pizza	Cheese Stuffed Turkey Meatballs	Pork Quesadillas	Beef chipotle	Spicy Lamb Meatballs with Mango Salsa	Sweet Potato Jackets	Chocolate Cake
Meal 2	Blueberry Cheesecake	Veggie Stuffed Peppers	Lamb Steak with Sweet Potatoes	Sticky Lemon Drumsticks	Apricot Glazed Turkey Legs	Honey Mustard Pork Chops	Spaghetti Meatballs on Stick
Meal 3	BBQ Pulled Pork with Coleslaw	Beef Kabobs	Classic Falafel	Vegetable Sushi	Tandoori Masala Chicken	Pistachio Stuffed Turkey Breast	Sweet and Sour Lamb Ribs

WEEK 40	Monday	Tuesday	Wednesday	Thursday	Friday	saturday	sunday
Meal 1	Mexican Chicken Wrap	Turkey Pattie with Avocado Salad	Crispy Coconut Pork Belly	Beef Stuffed Capsicum	Roasted Lamb Leg	Vegan Burrito Bowl	Pineapple Bites
Meal 2	Coconut Cookies	Cheesy Jalapenos	Lemon Herb Lamb Chops	Chicken Sandwich	Lemon Garlic Turkey	Balsamic Pork	Chinese beef and Broccoli
Meal 3	Salted beef with Caramelized Onions	Buffalo Cauliflower Wings	Turkey Meatloaf	Chocolate Fudge Brownies	Chicken Nuggets	Classic Lamb Shanks	BBQ Pork Sandwich

41	Monday	Tuesday	Wednesday	Thursday	Friday	saturday	sunday
Meal 1	Rotisserie Chicken	Turkey Burgers	Pork Dumplings	Chicken Lollipops	Beef and Mushroom Meatloaf	Skirt Steak Fajitas Wraps	Basil Lamb Cutlets
Meal 2	Blooming Onion with Spicy dip	Assorted Donuts	Tofu Satay	Sweet and Sour Cauliflower Stir fry	Eggplant Pizza	Sticky BBQ Tofu	Thai Beef Salad
Meal3	Herb Crusted Pork Ribs	Turkish Kebabs with Tahini Sauce	Butter-Honey Glazed Turkey	Thai Lamb Stir Fry	Buttery Pork Chops	Cranberry Turkey Wings	Thai Chicken Skewers

WEEK 42	Monday	Tuesday	Wednesday	Thursday	Friday	saturday	sunday
Meal 1	Beef with Mix Vegetables	Roasted Lamb Leg	Crispy Mongolian Beef	Potato Croquettes	Mediterranean Lamb Burgers	Sticky BBQ Honey Strips	Lamb Pie
Meal 2	Crispy Garlic Chicken with Lemon Dip	Black Bean Burger	Roasted Almond Chicken	Cinnamon Sugar Churros	Chicken Pie	Chocolate Soufflé	Vegetable Lasagna
Meal3	Kale chips	Turkey Sausages	Pork Medallions with Sour Cream	Turkey Quesadilla	Pork Steaks with Broccoli	Pineapple Turkey Kabobs	Pork Shoulder Skewers with Pineapple

WEEK 43	Monday	Tuesday	Wednesday	Thursday	Friday	saturday	sunday
Meal 1	Vegetable Spring rolls	Vegan Tacos	Cheesy Zucchini boat	Teriyaki Beef Steak with Broccoli	Chocolate Cake	Vegetable Fritters	Tropical Egg Rolls
Meal 2	Chicken Wings	Mexican Turkey Tacos	Lemon Pork Ribs	BBQ Chicken Pizza	Crispy Cheesy Lamb Chops	Beef chipotle	Plum Roast Lamb
Meal3	Crispy Pork	Walnut-Stuffed Lamb	Lemon Herb Beef Roast	Cheese Stuffed Turkey Meatballs	Honey Mustard Pork Chops	Almond Stuffed Chicken	Pulled Turkey Sandwich

WEEK 44	Monday	Tuesday	Wednesday	Thursday	Friday	saturday	sunday
Meal 1	Sticky Lemon Drumsticks	Apricot Glazed Turkey Legs	Pork Quesadillas	Spaghetti Meatballs on Stick	Spicy Lamb Meatballs with Mango Salsa	Beef Stuffed Capsicum	Turkey Pattie with Avocado Salad
Meal 2	Blueberry Cheesecake	Classic Falafel	Coconut Cookies	Sweet Potato Jackets	Veggie Stuffed Peppers	Chicken Sandwich	Vegan Burrito Bowl
Meal3	Lamb Steak with Sweet Potatoes	Crispy Coconut Pork Belly	Roasted Lamb Leg	Mexican Chicken Wrap	Lemon Garlic Turkey	Balsamic Pork	Chinese beef and Broccoli

WEEK 45	Monday	Tuesday	Wednesday	Thursday	Friday	saturday	sunday
Meal 1	Vegetable Sushi	Chicken Nuggets	Cheesy Jalapenos	Turkey Burgers	Blooming Onion with Spicy dip	BBQ Pork Sandwich	Sweet and Sour Cauliflower Stir fry
Meal 2	Butter-Honey Glazed Turkey	Pineapple Bites	Buttery Pork Chops	Salted beef with Caramelized Onions	Lemon Herb Lamb Chops	Chocolate Fudge Brownies	Sweet and Sour Lamb Ribs
Meal3	Thai Beef Salad	Classic Lamb Shanks	Beef Kabobs	Tandoori Masala Chicken	Herb Crusted Pork Ribs	Turkey Meatloaf	Thai Chicken Skewers

WEEK 46	Monday	Tuesday	Wednesday	Thursday	Friday	saturday	sunday
Meal 1	Chicken Lollipops	Cranberry Turkey Wings	Pork Dumplings	Skirt Steak Fajitas Wraps	Thai Lamb Stir Fry	Buffalo Cauliflower Wings	Sticky BBQ Tofu
Meal 2	Tofu Satay	Assorted Donuts	Crispy Garlic Chicken with Lemon Dip	Turkey Quesadilla	Kale chips	Beef and Mushroom Meatloaf	Roasted Lamb Leg
Meal 3	Pork Medallions with Sour Cream	Basil Lamb Cutlets	Chocolate Souffle	Almond Stuffed Chicken	Turkey Sausages	Crispy Pork	Beef with Mix Vegetables

WEEK 47	Monday	Tuesday	Wednesday	Thursday	Friday	saturday	sunday
Meal 1	Potato Croquettes	Black Bean Burger	Vegetable Spring rolls	Cinnamon Sugar Churros	Tropical Egg Rolls	Cheese Stuffed Turkey Meatballs	Rotisserie Chicken
Meal 2	Chicken Pie	Pulled Turkey Sandwich	Pork Steaks with Broccoli	Crispy Mongolian Beef	Lamb Pie	Eggplant Pizza	Lemon Pork Ribs
Meal 3	Teriyaki Beef Steak with Broccoli	Crispy Cheesy Lamb Chops	Sticky BBQ Honey Strips	Pineapple Turkey Kabobs	Roasted Almond Chicken	Pork Shoulder Skewers with Pineapple	Turkish Kebabs with Tahini Sauce

WEEK 48	Monday	Tuesday	Wednesday	Thursday	Friday	saturday	sunday
Meal 1	Chicken Wings	Pistachio Stuffed Turkey Breast	BBQ Pulled Pork with Coleslaw	Lemon Herb Beef Roast	Mediterranean Lamb Burgers	Vegetable Lasagna	Vegetable Fritters
Meal 2	Cheesy Zucchini boat	Plum Roast Lamb	BBQ Chicken Pizza	Mexican Turkey Tacos	Pork Quesadillas	Spaghetti Meatballs on Stick	Honey Mustard Pork Chops
Meal 3	Beef chipotle	Chocolate Cake	Veggie Stuffed Peppers	Coconut Cookies	Mexican Chicken Wrap	Apricot Glazed Turkey Legs	Spicy Lamb Meatballs with Mango Salsa

WEEK 49	Monday	Tuesday	Wednesday	Thursday	Friday	saturday	sunday
Meal 1	Tandoori Masala Chicken	Lemon Garlic Turkey	Sticky Lemon Drumsticks	Beef Stuffed Capsicum	Chicken Sandwich	Blooming Onion with Spicy dip	Turkey Pattie with Avocado Salad
Meal 2	Balsamic Pork	Chinese beef and Broccoli	BBQ Pork Sandwich	Turkey Meatloaf	Sweet and Sour Lamb Ribs	Blueberry Cheesecake	Walnut-Stuffed Lamb
Meal 3	Vegan Tacos	Lamb Steak with Sweet Potatoes	Classic Falafel	Beef Kabobs	Vegetable Sushi	Crispy Coconut Pork Belly	Raisin Bread Pudding with Chocolate

WEEK 50	Monday	Tuesday	Wednesday	Thursday	Friday	saturday	sunday
Meal 1	Chocolate Fudge Brownies	Butter-Honey Glazed Turkey	Buffalo Cauliflower Wings	Skirt Steak Fajitas Wraps	Assorted Donuts	Thai Chicken Skewers	Cheesy Jalapenos
Meal 2	Lemon Herb Lamb Chops	Pineapple Bites	Chicken Nuggets	Tofu Satay	Classic Lamb Shanks	Salted beef with Caramelized Onions	Turkey Burgers

Meal 3	Herb Crusted Pork Ribs	Thai Beef Salad	Roasted Lamb Leg	Pork Dumplings	Cranberry Turkey Wings	Buttery Pork Chops	Chicken Lollipops
	Herb Crusted Pork Ribs	Thai Beef Salad	Roasted Lamb Leg	Pork Dumplings	Cranberry Turkey Wings	Buttery Pork Chops	Chicken Lollipops

WEEK 51	Monday	Tuesday	Wednesday	Thursday	Friday	saturday	sunday
Meal 1	Teriyaki Beef Steak with Broccoli	Vegan Burrito Bowl	Thai Lamb Stir Fry	Coconut Cookies	Rotisserie Chicken	Mexican Turkey Tacos	Potato Croquettes
Meal 2	Pork Steaks with Broccoli	Pistachio Stuffed Turkey Breast	Roasted Almond Chicken	Beef chipotle	Basil Lamb Cutlets	Veggie Stuffed Peppers	Chocolate Soufflé
Meal 3	Chicken Wings	Lamb Pie	Pork Medallions with Sour Cream	Pineapple Turkey Kabobs	Black Bean Burger	Spaghetti Meatballs on Stick	BBQ Pulled Pork with Coleslaw

WEEK 52	Monday	Tuesday	Wednesday	Thursday	Friday	saturday	sunday
Meal 1	Mediterranean Lamb Burgers	Turkey Quesadilla	Pork Shoulder Skewers with Pineapple	Lemon Herb Beef Roast	Chicken Pie	Eggplant Pizza	Chocolate Cake
Meal 2	Cinnamon Sugar Churros	Mexican Chicken Wrap	Spicy Lamb Meatballs with Mango Salsa	Kale chips	Apricot Glazed Turkey Legs	Sticky BBQ Honey Strips	Crispy Pork
Meal 3	Beef with Mix Vegetables	Cheesy Zucchini boat	Sticky BBQ Tofu	Crispy Garlic Chicken with Lemon Dip	Turkish Kebabs with Tahini Sauce	Lemon Pork Ribs	Turkey Sausages

WEEK 53	Monday	Tuesday	Wednesday	Thursday	Friday	saturday	sunday
Meal 1	Pork Quesadillas	Vegetable Lasagna	Pulled Turkey Sandwich	Crispy Mongolian Beef	Plum Roast Lamb	Tandoori Masala Chicken	Tropical Egg Rolls
Meal 2	Almond Stuffed Chicken	Sweet and Sour Cauliflower Stir fry	Lamb Steak with Sweet Potatoes	Vegetable Spring rolls	Lemon Garlic Turkey	Balsamic Pork	Crispy Cheesy Lamb Chops
Meal 3	Beef Stuffed Capsicum	Honey Mustard Pork Chops	BBQ Chicken Pizza	Cheese Stuffed Turkey Meatballs	Vegetable Fritters	Sweet Potato Jackets	Beef and Mushroom Meatloaf

WEEK 54	Monday	Tuesday	Wednesday	Thursday	Friday	saturday	sunday
Meal 1	Skirt Steak Fajitas Wraps	Chicken Nuggets	BBQ Pork Sandwich	Blooming Onion with Spicy dip	Sweet and Sour Lamb Ribs	Turkey Pattie with Avocado Salad	Raisin Bread Pudding with Chocolate
Meal 2	Butter-Honey Glazed Turkey	Chocolate Fudge Brownies	Cheesy Jalapenos	Chicken Wings	Teriyaki Beef Steak with Broccoli	Buttery Pork Chops	Roasted Lamb Leg
Meal 3	Vegan Burrito Bowl	Thai Lamb Stir Fry	Lemon Garlic Turkey	BBQ Pulled Pork with Coleslaw	Coconut Cookies	Chinese beef and Broccoli	Sticky Lemon Drumsticks

WEEK 55	Monday	Tuesday	Wednesday	Thursday	Friday	saturday	sunday
Meal 1	Vegetable Sushi	Thai Chicken Skewers	Crispy Coconut Pork Belly	Salted beef with Caramelized Onions	Turkey Meatloaf	Blueberry Cheesecake	Basil Lamb Cutlets
Meal 2	Assorted Donuts	Cranberry Turkey Wings	Buffalo Cauliflower Wings	Chicken Sandwich	Lemon Herb Lamb Chops	Pork Medallions with Sour Cream	Beef chipotle
Meal 3	Herb Crusted Pork Ribs	Walnut-Stuffed Lamb	Chocolate Soufflé	Pineapple Turkey Kabobs	Beef Kabobs	Rotisserie Chicken	Veggie Stuffed Peppers

56	Monday	Tuesday	Wednesday	Thursday	Friday	saturday	sunday
Meal 1	Chicken Lollipops	Turkey Burgers	Pork Dumplings	Thai Beef Salad	Lamb Pie	Vegan Tacos	Classic Falafel
Meal 2	Pork Steaks with Broccoli	Tofu Satay	Crispy Garlic Chicken with Lemon Dip	Mediterranean Lamb Burgers	Pineapple Bites	Spaghetti Meatballs on Stick	Mexican Turkey Tacos
Meal 3	Black Bean Burger	Classic Lamb Shanks	Potato Croquettes	Turkey Quesadilla	Roasted Almond Chicken	Lemon Herb Beef Roast	Pork Shoulder Skewers with Pineapple

WEEK 57	Monday	Tuesday	Wednesday	Thursday	Friday	saturday	sunday
Meal 1	Chicken Pie	Pistachio Stuffed Turkey Breast	Crispy Pork	Sticky BBQ Honey Strips	Spicy Lamb Meatballs with Mango Salsa	Eggplant Pizza	Chocolate Cake
Meal 2	Cinnamon Sugar Churros	Kale chips	Mexican Chicken Wrap	Apricot Glazed Turkey Legs	Lemon Pork Ribs	Beef with Mix Vegetables	Turkish Kebabs with Tahini Sauce
Meal 3	Plum Roast Lamb	Crispy Mongolian Beef	Vegetable Lasagna	Pork Quesadillas	Tropical Egg Rolls	Pulled Turkey Sandwich	BBQ Chicken Pizza

WEEK 58	Monday	Tuesday	Wednesday	Thursday	Friday	saturday	sunday
Meal 1	Cheesy Zucchini boat	Vegetable Spring rolls	Sweet Potato Jackets	Sticky BBQ Tofu	Sweet and Sour Cauliflower Stir fry	Vegetable Fritters	Chicken Wings
Meal 2	Tandoori Masala Chicken	Cheese Stuffed Turkey Meatballs	Balsamic Pork	Beef Stuffed Capsicum	Lamb Steak with Sweet Potatoes	Almond Stuffed Chicken	Turkey Sausages
Meal 3	Chinese beef and Broccoli	Sweet and Sour Lamb Ribs	Crispy Cheesy Lamb Chops	Lemon Garlic Turkey	Honey Mustard Pork Chops	Beef and Mushroom Meatloaf	BBQ Pork Sandwich

WEEK 59	Monday	Tuesday	Wednesday	Thursday	Friday	saturday	sunday
Meal 1	Sticky Lemon Drumsticks	Skirt Steak Fajitas Wraps	Turkey Meatloaf	Blooming Onion with Spicy dip	Thai Lamb Stir Fry	Vegan Burrito Bowl	Chicken Nuggets
Meal 2	BBQ Pulled Pork with Coleslaw	Coconut Cookies	Assorted Donuts	Crispy Coconut Pork Belly	Chocolate Fudge Brownies	Beef Kabobs	Walnut-Stuffed Lamb
Meal 3	Cranberry Turkey Wings	Chicken Sandwich	Roasted Lamb Leg	Thai Beef Salad	Lemon Garlic Turkey	Buttery Pork Chops	Buffalo Cauliflower Wings

WEEK 60	Monday	Tuesday	Wednesday	Thursday	Friday	saturday	sunday
Meal 1	Raisin Bread Pudding with Chocolate	Turkey Pattie with Avocado Salad	Pork Dumplings	Cheesy Jalapenos	Thai Chicken Skewers	Vegetable Sushi	Salted beef with Caramelized Onions
Meal 2	Chicken Lollipops	Chocolate Soufflé	Veggie Stuffed Peppers	Spaghetti Meatballs on Stick	Pork Medallions with Sour Cream	Turkey Burgers	Blueberry Cheesecake
Meal 3	Herb Crusted Pork Ribs	Classic Lamb Shanks	Chicken Pie	Pineapple Turkey Kabobs	Spicy Lamb Meatballs with Mango Salsa	Teriyaki Beef Steak with Broccoli	Lemon Herb Lamb Chops

WEEK 61	Monday	Tuesday	Wednesday	Thursday	Friday	saturday	sunday
Meal 1	Eggplant Pizza	Sticky BBQ Tofu	Pork Steaks with Broccoli	Cheesy Zucchini boat	Basil Lamb Cutlets	Vegan Tacos	Beef chipotle
Meal 2	Roasted Almond Chicken	Mexican Turkey Tacos	Lamb Pie	Pistachio Stuffed Turkey Breast	Chocolate Cake	Crispy Pork	Classic Falafel
Meal 3	Pork Shoulder Skewers with Pineapple	Turkish Kebabs with Tahini Sauce	Mexican Chicken Wrap	Sticky BBQ Honey Strips	Rotisserie Chicken	Lemon Herb Beef Roast	Butter-Honey Glazed Turkey

WEEK 62	Monday	Tuesday	Wednesday	Thursday	Friday	saturday	sunday
Meal 1	Chinese beef and Broccoli	Cinnamon Sugar Churros	Crispy Garlic Chicken with Lemon Dip	Honey Mustard Pork Chops	Tofu Satay	Sweet and Sour Lamb Ribs	Sweet and Sour Cauliflower Stir fry
Meal 2	BBQ Chicken Pizza	Turkey Quesadilla	Pork Quesadillas	Beef with Mix Vegetables	Mediterranean Lamb Burgers	Kale chips	Crispy Mongolian Beef
Meal 3	Lemon Pork Ribs	Plum Roast Lamb	Vegetable Spring rolls	Pineapple Bites	Lemon Garlic Turkey	Almond Stuffed Chicken	Apricot Glazed Turkey Legs

WEEK 63	Monday	Tuesday	Wednesday	Thursday	Friday	saturday	sunday
Meal 1	Sweet Potato Jackets	Vegetable Fritters	Chicken Wings	Turkey Sausages	Balsamic Pork	Thai Beef Salad	Thai Lamb Stir Fry
Meal 2	BBQ Pulled Pork with Coleslaw	Sticky Lemon Drumsticks	Cheese Stuffed Turkey Meatballs	Lamb Steak with Sweet Potatoes	Beef Stuffed Capsicum	Tropical Egg Rolls	Vegetable Lasagna
Meal 3	Tandoori Masala Chicken	Pulled Turkey Sandwich	BBQ Pork Sandwich	Beef and Mushroom Meatloaf	Crispy Cheesy Lamb Chops	Potato Croquettes	Black Bean Burger

WEEK 64	Monday	Tuesday	Wednesday	Thursday	Friday	saturday	sunday
Meal 1	Chicken Nuggets	Turkey Meatloaf	Buttery Pork Chops	Skirt Steak Fajitas Wraps	Lemon Herb Lamb Chops	Blooming Onion with Spicy dip	Chocolate Fudge Brownies
Meal 2	Cheesy Jalapenos	Raisin Bread Pudding with Chocolate	Rotisserie Chicken	Turkey Pattie with Avocado Salad	Crispy Coconut Pork Belly	Teriyaki Beef Steak with Broccoli	Walnut-Stuffed Lamb
Meal 3	Beef chipotle	Roasted Lamb Leg	Vegan Tacos	Classic Falafel	Thai Chicken Skewers	Butter-Honey Glazed Turkey	Herb Crusted Pork Ribs

WEEK 65	Monday	Tuesday	Wednesday	Thursday	Friday	saturday	sunday
Meal 1	Coconut Cookies	Vegan Burrito Bowl	Basil Lamb Cutlets	Chicken Sandwich	Pork Medallions with Sour Cream	Cranberry Turkey Wings	Salted beef with Caramelized Onions
Meal 2	Roasted Almond Chicken	Pineapple Turkey Kabobs	Pork Steaks with Broccoli	Lemon Herb Beef Roast	Mediterranean Lamb Burgers	Vegetable Sushi	Blueberry Cheesecake
Meal 3	Lemon Pork Ribs	Chocolate Cake	Chicken Lollipops	Mexican Turkey Tacos	Eggplant Pizza	Beef Kabobs	Classic Lamb Shanks

WEEK 66	Monday	Tuesday	Wednesday	Thursday	Friday	saturday	sunday
Meal 1	Chicken Pie	Turkey Burgers	Pork Dumplings	Spaghetti Meatballs on Stick	Sticky BBQ Tofu	Buffalo Cauliflower Wings	Spicy Lamb Meatballs with Mango Salsa
Meal 2	Veggie Stuffed Peppers	Assorted Donuts	Cheesy Zucchini boat	Mexican Chicken Wrap	Pork Quesadillas	Lamb Pie	Chocolate Soufflé
Meal3	Pork Shoulder Skewers with Pineapple	Beef with Mix Vegetables	Crispy Garlic Chicken with Lemon Dip	Plum Roast Lamb	Pistachio Stuffed Turkey Breast	Sticky BBQ Honey Strips	Apricot Glazed Turkey Legs

WEEK 67	Monday	Tuesday	Wednesday	Thursday	Friday	saturday	sunday
Meal 1	BBQ Chicken Pizza	Turkey Quesadilla	Crispy Pork	Crispy Mongolian Beef	Turkish Kebabs with Tahini Sauce	Tofu Satay	Black Bean Burger
Meal 2	Sweet Potato Jackets	Pineapple Bites	Almond Stuffed Chicken	Lemon Garlic Turkey	Honey Mustard Pork Chops	Chinese beef and Broccoli	Sweet and Sour Lamb Ribs
Meal3	Thai Beef Salad	Thai Lamb Stir Fry	Potato Croquettes	Tropical Egg Rolls	Sticky Lemon Drumsticks	Pulled Turkey Sandwich	BBQ Pulled Pork with Coleslaw

WEEK 68	Monday	Tuesday	Wednesday	Thursday	Friday	saturday	sunday
Meal 1	Cinnamon Sugar Churros	Vegetable Spring rolls	Crispy Cheesy Lamb Chops	Beef and Mushroom Meatloaf	Balsamic Pork	Turkey Sausages	Chicken Wings
Meal 2	Lamb Steak with Sweet Potatoes	Beef Stuffed Capsicum	BBQ Pork Sandwich	Cheese Stuffed Turkey Meatballs	Chicken Nuggets	Sweet and Sour Cauliflower Stir fry	Kale chips
Meal3	Butter-Honey Glazed Turkey	Tandoori Masala Chicken	Vegetable Fritters	Vegetable Lasagna	Lemon Herb Lamb Chops	Teriyaki Beef Steak with Broccoli	Herb Crusted Pork Ribs

WEEK 69	Monday	Tuesday	Wednesday	Thursday	Friday	saturday	sunday
Meal 1	Thai Chicken Skewers	Turkey Meatloaf	Buttery Pork Chops	Skirt Steak Fajitas Wraps	Spicy Lamb Meatballs with Mango Salsa	Blooming Onion with Spicy dip	Chocolate Fudge Brownies
Meal 2	Classic Lamb Shanks	Vegan Burrito Bowl	Coconut Cookies	Chicken Sandwich	Cranberry Turkey Wings	Pork Medallions with Sour Cream	Beef Kabobs
Meal3	Turkey Burgers	Pork Dumplings	Spaghetti Meatballs on Stick	Roasted Lamb Leg	Buffalo Cauliflower Wings	Blueberry Cheesecake	Chicken Pie

WEEK 70	Monday	Tuesday	Wednesday	Thursday	Friday	saturday	sunday
Meal 1	Rotisserie Chicken	Turkey Pattie with Avocado Salad	Crispy Coconut Pork Belly	Beef chipotle	Walnut-Stuffed Lamb	Cheesy Jalapenos	Raisin Bread Pudding with Chocolate
Meal 2	Salted beef with Caramelized Onions	Basil Lamb Cutlets	Vegetable Sushi	Classic Falafel	Chicken Lollipops	Pineapple Turkey Kabobs	Pork Steaks with Broccoli
Meal3	Veggie Stuffed Peppers	Chocolate Cake	Mexican Chicken Wrap	Pistachio Stuffed Turkey Breast	Pork Shoulder Skewers with Pineapple	Sticky BBQ Honey Strips	Lamb Pie

WEEK 71	Monday	Tuesday	Wednesday	Thursday	Friday	saturday	sunday
Meal 1	Roasted Almond Chicken	Mexican Turkey Tacos	Lemon Pork Ribs	Lemon Herb Beef Roast	Mediterranean Lamb Burgers	Vegan Tacos	Assorted Donuts
Meal 2	Beef with Mix Vegetables	Plum Roast Lamb	Eggplant Pizza	Pineapple Bites	Crispy Garlic Chicken with Lemon Dip	Apricot Glazed Turkey Legs	Pork Quesadillas
Meal 3	Cheesy Zucchini boat	Cinnamon Sugar Churros	Chicken Nuggets	Turkey Quesadilla	Crispy Pork	Crispy Mongolian Beef	Turkish Kebabs with Tahini Sauce

72	Monday	Tuesday	Wednesday	Thursday	Friday	saturday	sunday
Meal 1	Chicken Wings	Lemon Garlic Turkey	Honey Mustard Pork Chops	Chinese beef and Broccoli	Sweet and Sour Lamb Ribs	Tofu Satay	Chocolate Soufflé
Meal 2	Vegetable Spring rolls	Black Bean Burger	Tandoori Masala Chicken	Cheese Stuffed Turkey Meatballs	Balsamic Pork	Beef and Mushroom Meatloaf	Crispy Cheesy Lamb Chops
Meal 3	Beef Stuffed Capsicum	Lamb Steak with Sweet Potatoes	Vegetable Lasagna	Sweet and Sour Cauliflower Stir fry	BBQ Chicken Pizza	Butter-Honey Glazed Turkey	BBQ Pork Sandwich

WEEK 73	Monday	Tuesday	Wednesday	Thursday	Friday	saturday	sunday
Meal 1	Almond Stuffed Chicken	Pulled Turkey Sandwich	Buttery Pork Chops	Thai Beef Salad	Thai Lamb Stir Fry	Sweet Potato Jackets	Sticky BBQ Tofu
Meal 2	Potato Croquettes	Tropical Egg Rolls	Sticky Lemon Drumsticks	Turkey Sausages	BBQ Pulled Pork with Coleslaw	Teriyaki Beef Steak with Broccoli	Lemon Herb Lamb Chops
Meal 3	Skirt Steak Fajitas Wraps	Roasted Lamb Leg	Kale chips	Vegetable Fritters	Thai Chicken Skewers	Turkey Meatloaf	Herb Crusted Pork Ribs

WEEK 74	Monday	Tuesday	Wednesday	Thursday	Friday	saturday	sunday
Meal 1	Chicken Sandwich	Cranberry Turkey Wings	Pork Medallions with Sour Cream	Beef Kabobs	Classic Lamb Shanks	Blooming Onion with Spicy dip	Chocolate Fudge Brownies
Meal 2	Cheesy Jalapenos	Raisin Bread Pudding with Chocolate	Rotisserie Chicken	Pineapple Turkey Kabobs	Pork Steaks with Broccoli	Salted beef with Caramelized Onions	Basil Lamb Cutlets
Meal 3	Beef with Mix Vegetables	Plum Roast Lamb	Vegan Tacos	Assorted Donuts	Roasted Almond Chicken	Apricot Glazed Turkey Legs	Pork Quesadillas

WEEK 75	Monday	Tuesday	Wednesday	Thursday	Friday	saturday	sunday
Meal 1	Coconut Cookies	Chicken Pie	Turkey Burgers	Pork Dumplings	Spaghetti Meatballs on Stick	Spicy Lamb Meatballs with Mango Salsa	Vegan Burrito Bowl
Meal 2	Lamb Pie	Vegetable Sushi	Classic Falafel	Chicken Lollipops	Pistachio Stuffed Turkey Breast	Pork Shoulder Skewers with Pineapple	Sticky BBQ Honey Strips
Meal 3	Crispy Pork	Crispy Mongolian Beef	Turkish Kebabs with Tahini Sauce	Tofu Satay	Chocolate Soufflé	Crispy Garlic Chicken with Lemon Dip	Turkey Quesadilla

98

WEEK 76	Monday	Tuesday	Wednesday	Thursday	Friday	saturday	sunday
Meal 1	Buffalo Cauliflower Wings	Mexican Chicken Wrap	Beef and Mushroom Meatloaf	Crispy Coconut Pork Belly	Turkey Pattie with Avocado Salad	Walnut-Stuffed Lamb	Blueberry Cheesecake
Meal 2	Mediterranean Lamb Burgers	Chocolate Cake	Veggie Stuffed Peppers	Chicken Nuggets	Beef Stuffed Capsicum	Lemon Pork Ribs	Mexican Turkey Tacos
Meal 3	Honey Mustard Pork Chops	Lemon Garlic Turkey	Sweet and Sour Lamb Ribs	Black Bean Burger	Vegetable Spring rolls	Tandoori Masala Chicken	Skirt Steak Fajitas Wraps

WEEK 77	Monday	Tuesday	Wednesday	Thursday	Friday	saturday	sunday
Meal 1	Eggplant Pizza	Crispy Cheesy Lamb Chops	Balsamic Pork	Cheese Stuffed Turkey Meatballs	Thai Beef Salad	Pineapple Bites	BBQ Chicken Pizza
Meal 2	Sweet and Sour Cauliflower Stir fry	Chicken Wings	Vegetable Lasagna	Lemon Herb Lamb Chops	BBQ Pulled Pork with Coleslaw	Pulled Turkey Sandwich	Teriyaki Beef Steak with Broccoli
Meal 3	Turkey Meatloaf	Beef Kabobs	Tropical Egg Rolls	Thai Chicken Skewers	Potato Croquettes	Roasted Lamb Leg	Buttery Pork Chops

WEEK 78	Monday	Tuesday	Wednesday	Thursday	Friday	saturday	sunday
Meal 1	Lamb Steak with Sweet Potatoes	Almond Stuffed Chicken	Beef chipotle	BBQ Pork Sandwich	Cheesy Zucchini boat	Butter-Honey Glazed Turkey	Cinnamon Sugar Churros
Meal 2	Turkey Sausages	Sticky BBQ Tofu	Thai Lamb Stir Fry	Sticky Lemon Drumsticks	Lemon Herb Beef Roast	Herb Crusted Pork Ribs	Sweet Potato Jackets
Meal 3	Pork Medallions with Sour Cream	Kale chips	Cranberry Turkey Wings	Vegetable Fritters	Classic Lamb Shanks	Chicken Sandwich	Chinese beef and Broccoli

WEEK 79	Monday	Tuesday	Wednesday	Thursday	Friday	saturday	sunday
Meal 1	Pork Steaks with Broccoli	Pineapple Turkey Kabobs	Basil Lamb Cutlets	Rotisserie Chicken	Salted beef with Caramelized Onions	Chocolate Fudge Brownies	Blooming Onion with Spicy dip
Meal 2	Classic Falafel	Vegetable Sushi	Pork Dumplings	Turkey Burgers	Spicy Lamb Meatballs with Mango Salsa	Chicken Pie	Spaghetti Meatballs on Stick
Meal 3	Mexican Chicken Wrap	Beef Stuffed Capsicum	Assorted Donuts	Vegan Tacos	Crispy Coconut Pork Belly	Turkey Pattie with Avocado Salad	Walnut-Stuffed Lamb

WEEK 80	Monday	Tuesday	Wednesday	Thursday	Friday	saturday	sunday
Meal 1	Cheesy Jalapenos	Beef with Mix Vegetables	Roasted Almond Chicken	Pork Quesadillas	Raisin Bread Pudding with Chocolate	Plum Roast Lamb	Apricot Glazed Turkey Legs
Meal 2	Lamb Pie	Pistachio Stuffed Turkey Breast	Vegan Burrito Bowl	Sticky BBQ Honey Strips	Chicken Lollipops	Pork Shoulder Skewers with Pineapple	Coconut Cookies
Meal 3	Honey Mustard Pork Chops	Blueberry Cheesecake	Sweet and Sour Lamb Ribs	Lemon Garlic Turkey	Buffalo Cauliflower Wings	Chinese beef and Broccoli	Chicken Nuggets

81	Monday	Tuesday	Wednesday	Thursday	Friday	saturday	sunday
Meal 1	Turkish Kebabs with Tahini Sauce	Crispy Garlic Chicken with Lemon Dip	Crispy Pork	Turkey Quesadilla	Tofu Satay	Crispy Mongolian Beef	Chocolate Soufflé
Meal 2	Eggplant Pizza	Beef and Mushroom Meatloaf	Pineapple Bites	Crispy Cheesy Lamb Chops	Tandoori Masala Chicken	Balsamic Pork	Cheese Stuffed Turkey Meatballs
Meal3	BBQ Chicken Pizza	BBQ Pulled Pork with Coleslaw	Pulled Turkey Sandwich	Cheesy Zucchini boat	Beef chipotle	Cinnamon Sugar Churros	Lemon Herb Lamb Chops

WEEK 82	Monday	Tuesday	Wednesday	Thursday	Friday	saturday	sunday
Meal 1	Chicken Wings	Mexican Turkey Tacos	Lemon Pork Ribs	Lemon Herb Beef Roast	Mediterranean Lamb Burgers	Veggie Stuffed Peppers	Chocolate Cake
Meal 2	Thai Lamb Stir Fry	Vegetable Lasagna	Sweet and Sour Cauliflower Stir fry	Almond Stuffed Chicken	Turkey Sausages	Herb Crusted Pork Ribs	Teriyaki Beef Steak with Broccoli
Meal3	Cranberry Turkey Wings	Pork Medallions with Sour Cream	Beef Kabobs	Classic Lamb Shanks	Sweet Potato Jackets	Sticky BBQ Tofu	Chicken Sandwich

WEEK 83	Monday	Tuesday	Wednesday	Thursday	Friday	saturday	sunday
Meal 1	Skirt Steak Fajitas Wraps	Thai Chicken Skewers	Vegetable Spring rolls	Buttery Pork Chops	Black Bean Burger	Roasted Lamb Leg	Turkey Meatloaf
Meal 2	Tropical Egg Rolls	Lamb Steak with Sweet Potatoes	Butter-Honey Glazed Turkey	Thai Beef Salad	Sticky Lemon Drumsticks	Potato Croquettes	BBQ Pork Sandwich
Meal3	Kale chips	Pork Steaks with Broccoli	Vegetable Fritters	Basil Lamb Cutlets	Pineapple Turkey Kabobs	Salted beef with Caramelized Onions	Rotisserie Chicken

WEEK 84	Monday	Tuesday	Wednesday	Thursday	Friday	saturday	sunday
Meal 1	Chicken Pie	Turkey Burgers	Pork Dumplings	Spaghetti Meatballs on Stick	Spicy Lamb Meatballs with Mango Salsa	Vegetable Sushi	Classic Falafel
Meal 2	Cheesy Jalapenos	Raisin Bread Pudding with Chocolate	Roasted Almond Chicken	Apricot Glazed Turkey Legs	Pork Quesadillas	Beef with Mix Vegetables	Plum Roast Lamb
Meal3	Turkish Kebabs with Tahini Sauce	Tofu Satay	Chocolate Soufflé	Crispy Garlic Chicken with Lemon Dip	Turkey Quesadilla	Crispy Pork	Crispy Mongolian Beef

WEEK 85	Monday	Tuesday	Wednesday	Thursday	Friday	saturday	sunday
Meal 1	Chicken Lollipops	Pistachio Stuffed Turkey Breast	Pork Shoulder Skewers with Pineapple	Beef Stuffed Capsicum	Lamb Pie	Blooming Onion with Spicy dip	Chocolate Fudge Brownies
Meal 2	Crispy Cheesy Lamb Chops	Vegan Burrito Bowl	Coconut Cookies	Tandoori Masala Chicken	Cheese Stuffed Turkey Meatballs	Balsamic Pork	Sticky BBQ Honey Strips
Meal3	Mexican Turkey Tacos	Lemon Pork Ribs	Beef and Mushroom Meatloaf	Mediterranean Lamb Burgers	Cheesy Zucchini boat	Cinnamon Sugar Churros	Chicken Wings

WEEK 86	Monday	Tuesday	Wednesday	Thursday	Friday	saturday	sunday
Meal 1	Walnut-Stuffed Lamb	Vegan Tacos	Crispy Coconut Pork Belly	Chicken Nuggets	Lemon Garlic Turkey	Assorted Donuts	Chinese beef and Broccoli
Meal 2	Pulled Turkey Sandwich	Pineapple Bites	Beef chipotle	Sweet and Sour Lamb Ribs	Eggplant Pizza	Pork Medallions with Sour Cream	BBQ Chicken Pizza
Meal 3	Pork Steaks with Broccoli	Rotisserie Chicken	Pineapple Turkey Kabobs	Chocolate Cake	Salted beef with Caramelized Onions	Basil Lamb Cutlets	Veggie Stuffed Peppers

WEEK 87	Monday	Tuesday	Wednesday	Thursday	Friday	saturday	sunday
Meal 1	Honey Mustard Pork Chops	Blueberry Cheesecake	Turkey Sausages	Mexican Chicken Wrap	Lemon Herb Beef Roast	Buffalo Cauliflower Wings	Lemon Herb Lamb Chops
Meal 2	Vegetable Spring rolls	Roasted Lamb Leg	BBQ Pulled Pork with Coleslaw	Tropical Egg Rolls	Cranberry Turkey Wings	Almond Stuffed Chicken	Skirt Steak Fajitas Wraps
Meal 3	Sticky Lemon Drumsticks	Thai Beef Salad	Potato Croquettes	Lamb Steak with Sweet Potatoes	Herb Crusted Pork Ribs	Vegetable Fritters	Butter-Honey Glazed Turkey

88	Monday	Tuesday	Wednesday	Thursday	Friday	saturday	sunday
Meal 1	Vegetable Lasagna	Sweet and Sour Cauliflower Stir fry	Turkey Pattie with Avocado Salad	Buttery Pork Chops	Chicken Sandwich	Teriyaki Beef Steak with Broccoli	Thai Lamb Stir Fry
Meal 2	Beef Kabobs	Classic Lamb Shanks	Sweet Potato Jackets	Sticky BBQ Tofu	Turkey Meatloaf	BBQ Pork Sandwich	Thai Chicken Skewers
Meal 3	Pork Dumplings	Chicken Pie	Spaghetti Meatballs on Stick	Plum Roast Lamb	Kale chips	Black Bean Burger	Turkey Burgers

WEEK 89	Monday	Tuesday	Wednesday	Thursday	Friday	saturday	sunday
Meal 1	Roasted Almond Chicken	Apricot Glazed Turkey Legs	Pork Quesadillas	Beef with Mix Vegetables	Spicy Lamb Meatballs with Mango Salsa	Vegetable Sushi	Classic Falafel
Meal 2	Blooming Onion with Spicy dip	Chocolate Fudge Brownies	Chicken Lollipops	Pistachio Stuffed Turkey Breast	Pork Shoulder Skewers with Pineapple	Beef Stuffed Capsicum	Lamb Pie
Meal 3	Chinese beef and Broccoli	Walnut-Stuffed Lamb	Vegan Tacos	Assorted Donuts	Chicken Nuggets	Lemon Garlic Turkey	Crispy Coconut Pork Belly

WEEK 90	Monday	Tuesday	Wednesday	Thursday	Friday	saturday	sunday
Meal 1	Turkey Quesadilla	Crispy Pork	Crispy Mongolian Beef	Turkish Kebabs with Tahini Sauce	Cheesy Jalapenos	Raisin Bread Pudding with Chocolate	Crispy Garlic Chicken with Lemon Dip
Meal 2	Coconut Cookies	Tandoori Masala Chicken	Cheese Stuffed Turkey Meatballs	Balsamic Pork	Sticky BBQ Honey Strips	Crispy Cheesy Lamb Chops	Vegan Burrito Bowl
Meal 3	Sweet and Sour Lamb Ribs	Eggplant Pizza	Pineapple Bites	BBQ Chicken Pizza	Pulled Turkey Sandwich	Pork Medallions with Sour Cream	Beef chipotle

WEEK 91	Monday	Tuesday	Wednesday	Thursday	Friday	saturday	sunday
Meal 1	Lemon Pork Ribs	Beef and Mushroom Meatloaf	Mediterranean Lamb Burgers	Tofu Satay	Chocolate Soufflé	Chicken Wings	Mexican Turkey Tacos
Meal 2	Rotisserie Chicken	Pineapple Turkey Kabobs	Pork Steaks with Broccoli	Salted beef with Caramelized Onions	Basil Lamb Cutlets	Sweet Potato Jackets	Sticky BBQ Tofu
Meal 3	Kale chips	Black Bean Burger	Chicken Pie	Turkey Pattie with Avocado Salad	Pork Dumplings	Spaghetti Meatballs on Stick	Plum Roast Lamb

WEEK 92	Monday	Tuesday	Wednesday	Thursday	Friday	saturday	sunday
Meal 1	Lemon Herb Beef Roast	Lemon Herb Lamb Chops	Cheesy Zucchini boat	Cinnamon Sugar Churros	Mexican Chicken Wrap	Butter-Honey Glazed Turkey	Honey Mustard Pork Chops
Meal 2	Turkey Meatloaf	Buttery Pork Chops	Teriyaki Beef Steak with Broccoli	Thai Lamb Stir Fry	Vegetable Spring rolls	Tropical Egg Rolls	Chicken Sandwich
Meal 3	Vegetable Fritters	Thai Chicken Skewers	Turkey Burgers	BBQ Pork Sandwich	Beef Kabobs	Classic Lamb Shanks	Potato Croquettes

WEEK 93	Monday	Tuesday	Wednesday	Thursday	Friday	saturday	sunday
Meal 1	Roasted Lamb Leg	Veggie Stuffed Peppers	Chocolate Cake	Almond Stuffed Chicken	Turkey Sausages	BBQ Pulled Pork with Coleslaw	Skirt Steak Fajitas Wraps
Meal 2	Herb Crusted Pork Ribs	Thai Beef Salad	Lamb Steak with Sweet Potatoes	Buffalo Cauliflower Wings	Blueberry Cheesecake	Sticky Lemon Drumsticks	Cranberry Turkey Wings
Meal 3	Roasted Almond Chicken	Apricot Glazed Turkey Legs	Pork Quesadillas	Beef with Mix Vegetables	Spicy Lamb Meatballs with Mango Salsa	Vegetable Lasagna	Sweet and Sour Cauliflower Stir fry

WEEK 94	Monday	Tuesday	Wednesday	Thursday	Friday	saturday	sunday
Meal 1	Vegetable Sushi	Classic Falafel	Chicken Lollipops	Pistachio Stuffed Turkey Breast	Pork Shoulder Skewers with Pineapple	Beef Stuffed Capsicum	Lamb Pie
Meal 2	Crispy Pork	Crispy Mongolian Beef	Turkish Kebabs with Tahini Sauce	Cheesy Jalapenos	Raisin Bread Pudding with Chocolate	Crispy Garlic Chicken with Lemon Dip	Turkey Quesadilla
Meal 3	Chocolate Soufflé	Chicken Wings	Mexican Turkey Tacos	Lemon Pork Ribs	Beef and Mushroom Meatloaf	Mediterranean Lamb Burgers	Tofu Satay

WEEK 95	Monday	Tuesday	Wednesday	Thursday	Friday	saturday	sunday
Meal 1	Chocolate Fudge Brownies	Chicken Nuggets	Lemon Garlic Turkey	Crispy Coconut Pork Belly	Chinese beef and Broccoli	Walnut-Stuffed Lamb	Blooming Onion with Spicy dip
Meal 2	Crispy Cheesy Lamb Chops	Vegan Burrito Bowl	Coconut Cookies	Tandoori Masala Chicken	Cheese Stuffed Turkey Meatballs	Balsamic Pork	Sticky BBQ Honey Strips
Meal 3	Pork Steaks with Broccoli	Salted beef with Caramelized Onions	Basil Lamb Cutlets	Sweet Potato Jackets	Sticky BBQ Tofu	Rotisserie Chicken	Pineapple Turkey Kabobs

116

96	Monday	Tuesday	Wednesday	Thursday	Friday	saturday	sunday
Meal 1	BBQ Chicken Pizza	Pulled Turkey Sandwich	Pork Medallions with Sour Cream	Beef chipotle	Sweet and Sour Lamb Ribs	Vegan Tacos	Assorted Donuts
Meal 2	Cheesy Zucchini boat	Cinnamon Sugar Churros	Chicken Pie	Turkey Pattie with Avocado Salad	Pork Dumplings	Spaghetti Meatballs on Stick	Plum Roast Lamb
Meal 3	Beef with Mix Vegetables	Spicy Lamb Meatballs with Mango Salsa	Veggie Stuffed Peppers	Chocolate Cake	Roasted Almond Chicken	Apricot Glazed Turkey Legs	Pork Quesadillas

WEEK 97	Monday	Tuesday	Wednesday	Thursday	Friday	saturday	sunday
Meal 1	Butter-Honey Glazed Turkey	Honey Mustard Pork Chops	Lemon Herb Beef Roast	Lemon Herb Lamb Chops	Eggplant Pizza	Pineapple Bites	Mexican Chicken Wrap
Meal 2	Black Bean Burger	Almond Stuffed Chicken	Turkey Sausages	BBQ Pulled Pork with Coleslaw	Skirt Steak Fajitas Wraps	Roasted Lamb Leg	Kale chips
Meal 3	Lamb Steak with Sweet Potatoes	Vegetable Lasagna	Sweet and Sour Cauliflower Stir fry	Sticky Lemon Drumsticks	Cranberry Turkey Wings	Herb Crusted Pork Ribs	Thai Beef Salad

WEEK 98	Monday	Tuesday	Wednesday	Thursday	Friday	saturday	sunday
Meal 1	Buttery Pork Chops	Teriyaki Beef Steak with Broccoli	Thai Lamb Stir Fry	Vegetable Spring rolls	Tropical Egg Rolls	Chicken Sandwich	Turkey Meatloaf
Meal 2	Thai Chicken Skewers	Turkey Burgers	BBQ Pork Sandwich	Beef Kabobs	Classic Lamb Shanks	Potato Croquettes	Vegetable Fritters
Meal 3	Buffalo Cauliflower Wings	Blueberry Cheesecake	Crispy Garlic Chicken with Lemon Dip	Pistachio Stuffed Turkey Breast	Pork Shoulder Skewers with Pineapple	Beef Stuffed Capsicum	Lamb Pie

WEEK 99	Monday	Tuesday	Wednesday	Thursday	Friday	saturday	sunday
Meal 1	Crispy Mongolian Beef	Turkish Kebabs with Tahini Sauce	Vegetable Sushi	Classic Falafel	Chicken Lollipops	Turkey Quesadilla	Crispy Pork
Meal 2	Cheese Stuffed Turkey Meatballs	Balsamic Pork	Sticky BBQ Honey Strips	Crispy Cheesy Lamb Chops	Blooming Onion with Spicy dip	Chocolate Fudge Brownies	Tandoori Masala Chicken
Meal 3	Assorted Donuts	BBQ Chicken Pizza	Pulled Turkey Sandwich	Pork Medallions with Sour Cream	Beef chipotle	Sweet and Sour Lamb Ribs	Vegan Tacos

WEEK 100	Monday	Tuesday	Wednesday	Thursday	Friday	saturday	sunday
Meal 1	Mediterranean Lamb Burgers	Cheesy Jalapenos	Raisin Bread Pudding with Chocolate	Chicken Wings	Mexican Turkey Tacos	Lemon Pork Ribs	Beef and Mushroom Meatloaf
Meal 2	Crispy Coconut Pork Belly	Chinese beef and Broccoli	Walnut-Stuffed Lamb	Vegan Burrito Bowl	Coconut Cookies	Chicken Nuggets	Lemon Garlic Turkey
Meal 3	Chicken Pie	Turkey Pattie with Avocado Salad	Pork Dumplings	Spaghetti Meatballs on Stick	Plum Roast Lamb	Cheesy Zucchini boat	Cinnamon Sugar Churros

WEEK 101	Monday	Tuesday	Wednesday	Thursday	Friday	saturday	sunday
Meal 1	Tofu Satay	Chocolate Soufflé	Rotisserie Chicken	Pineapple Turkey Kabobs	Pork Steaks with Broccoli	Salted beef with Caramelized Onions	Basil Lamb Cutlets
Meal 2	Beef with Mix Vegetables	Spicy Lamb Meatballs with Mango Salsa	Sweet Potato Jackets	Sticky BBQ Tofu	Roasted Almond Chicken	Apricot Glazed Turkey Legs	Pork Quesadillas
Meal3	Pistachio Stuffed Turkey Breast	Pork Shoulder Skewers with Pineapple	Beef Stuffed Capsicum	Lamb Pie	Vegetable Spring rolls	Tropical Egg Rolls	Crispy Garlic Chicken with Lemon Dip

102	Monday	Tuesday	Wednesday	Thursday	Friday	saturday	sunday
Meal 1	Chocolate Cake	Mexican Chicken Wrap	Butter-Honey Glazed Turkey	Honey Mustard Pork Chops	Lemon Herb Beef Roast	Lemon Herb Lamb Chops	Veggie Stuffed Peppers
Meal 2	Thai Lamb Stir Fry	Eggplant Pizza	Pineapple Bites	Chicken Sandwich	Turkey Meatloaf	Buttery Pork Chops	Teriyaki Beef Steak with Broccoli
Meal3	BBQ Pork Sandwich	Beef Kabobs	Classic Lamb Shanks	Potato Croquettes	Vegetable Fritters	Thai Chicken Skewers	Turkey Burgers

WEEK 103	Monday	Tuesday	Wednesday	Thursday	Friday	saturday	sunday
Meal 1	Skirt Steak Fajitas Wraps	Kale chips	Turkey Sausages	Black Bean Burger	Roasted Lamb Leg	Almond Stuffed Chicken	BBQ Pulled Pork with Coleslaw
Meal 2	Sticky Lemon Drumsticks	Herb Crusted Pork Ribs	Thai Beef Salad	Vegetable Lasagna	Cranberry Turkey Wings	Sweet and Sour Cauliflower Stir fry	Lamb Steak with Sweet Potatoes
Meal3	Blueberry Cheesecake	Turkish Kebabs with Tahini Sauce	Chicken Lollipops	Crispy Pork	Crispy Mongolian Beef	Buffalo Cauliflower Wings	Turkey Quesadilla

WEEK 104	Monday	Tuesday	Wednesday	Thursday	Friday	saturday	sunday
Meal 1	Tandoori Masala Chicken	Cheese Stuffed Turkey Meatballs	Balsamic Pork	Sticky BBQ Honey Strips	Crispy Cheesy Lamb Chops	Vegetable Sushi	Classic Falafel
Meal 2	Cheesy Jalapenos	Raisin Bread Pudding with Chocolate	Chicken Wings	Mexican Turkey Tacos	Lemon Pork Ribs	Beef and Mushroom Meatloaf	Mediterranean Lamb Burgers
Meal3	Salted beef with Caramelized Onions	Basil Lamb Cutlets	Tofu Satay	Chocolate Soufflé	Rotisserie Chicken	Pineapple Turkey Kabobs	Pork Steaks with Broccoli

WEEK 105	Monday	Tuesday	Wednesday	Thursday	Friday	saturday	sunday
Meal 1	Beef chipotle	BBQ Chicken Pizza	Pork Medallions with Sour Cream	Pulled Turkey Sandwich	Sweet and Sour Lamb Ribs	Chocolate Fudge Brownies	Blooming Onion with Spicy dip
Meal 2	Spicy Lamb Meatballs with Mango Salsa	Coconut Cookies	Vegan Burrito Bowl	Beef with Mix Vegetables	Roasted Almond Chicken	Pork Quesadillas	Apricot Glazed Turkey Legs
Meal3	Mexican Chicken Wrap	Honey Mustard Pork Chops	Butter-Honey Glazed Turkey	Lemon Herb Lamb Chops	Pineapple Bites	Eggplant Pizza	Lemon Herb Beef Roast

104

WEEK 106	Monday	Tuesday	Wednesday	Thursday	Friday	saturday	sunday
Meal 1	Vegan Tacos	Lemon Garlic Turkey	Blueberry Cheesecake	Chinese beef and Broccoli	Chicken Nuggets	Crispy Coconut Pork Belly	Walnut-Stuffed Lamb
Meal 2	Crispy Garlic Chicken with Lemon Dip	Buttery Pork Chops	Lamb Pie	Kale chips	Pistachio Stuffed Turkey Breast	Assorted Donuts	Beef Stuffed Capsicum
Meal 3	Turkey Quesadilla	Black Bean Burger	Crispy Mongolian Beef	Chicken Lollipops	Crispy Pork	Turkish Kebabs with Tahini Sauce	Buffalo Cauliflower Wings

WEEK 107	Monday	Tuesday	Wednesday	Thursday	Friday	saturday	sunday
Meal 1	Cinnamon Sugar Churros	Turkey Meatloaf	Spaghetti Meatballs on Stick	Pork Shoulder Skewers with Pineapple	Chicken Pie	Cheesy Zucchini boat	Plum Roast Lamb
Meal 2	Sweet Potato Jackets	Roasted Lamb Leg	Sticky BBQ Tofu	Turkey Sausages	Skirt Steak Fajitas Wraps	BBQ Pulled Pork with Coleslaw	Almond Stuffed Chicken
Meal 3	Herb Crusted Pork Ribs	Sticky Lemon Drumsticks	Vegetable Lasagna	Lamb Steak with Sweet Potatoes	Sweet and Sour Cauliflower Stir fry	Cranberry Turkey Wings	Thai Beef Salad

WEEK 108	Monday	Tuesday	Wednesday	Thursday	Friday	saturday	sunday
Meal 1	Chicken Sandwich	Turkey Pattie with Avocado Salad	Pork Dumplings	Teriyaki Beef Steak with Broccoli	Thai Lamb Stir Fry	Vegetable Spring rolls	Tropical Egg Rolls
Meal 2	Veggie Stuffed Peppers	Chocolate Cake	Thai Chicken Skewers	Turkey Burgers	BBQ Pork Sandwich	Beef Kabobs	Classic Lamb Shanks
Meal 3	Sticky BBQ Honey Strips	Mediterranean Lamb Burgers	Potato Croquettes	Vegetable Fritters	Chicken Wings	Cheese Stuffed Turkey Meatballs	Balsamic Pork

WEEK 109	Monday	Tuesday	Wednesday	Thursday	Friday	saturday	sunday
Meal 1	Salted beef with Caramelized Onions	Mexican Turkey Tacos	Pork Steaks with Broccoli	Classic Falafel	Tandoori Masala Chicken	Vegetable Sushi	Basil Lamb Cutlets
Meal 2	Blooming Onion with Spicy dip	Sweet and Sour Lamb Ribs	Beef chipotle	Apricot Glazed Turkey Legs	Pork Medallions with Sour Cream	Chocolate Fudge Brownies	BBQ Chicken Pizza
Meal 3	Blueberry Cheesecake	Crispy Garlic Chicken with Lemon Dip	Buffalo Cauliflower Wings	Walnut-Stuffed Lamb	Chinese beef and Broccoli	Lemon Garlic Turkey	Crispy Coconut Pork Belly

WEEK 110	Monday	Tuesday	Wednesday	Thursday	Friday	saturday	sunday
Meal 1	Pineapple Turkey Kabobs	Rotisserie Chicken	Lemon Pork Ribs	Raisin Bread Pudding with Chocolate	Crispy Cheesy Lamb Chops	Cheesy Jalapenos	Beef and Mushroom Meatloaf
Meal 2	Eggplant Pizza	Beef with Mix Vegetables	Pulled Turkey Sandwich	Mexican Chicken Wrap	Pork Quesadillas	Pineapple Bites	Spicy Lamb Meatballs with Mango Salsa
Meal 3	Assorted Donuts	Turkish Kebabs with Tahini Sauce	Vegan Tacos	Beef Stuffed Capsicum	Pistachio Stuffed Turkey Breast	Chicken Nuggets	Buttery Pork Chops

105

111	Monday	Tuesday	Wednesday	Thursday	Friday	saturday	sunday
Meal 1	Roasted Almond Chicken	Butter-Honey Glazed Turkey	Honey Mustard Pork Chops	Lemon Herb Beef Roast	Lemon Herb Lamb Chops	Vegan Burrito Bowl	Coconut Cookies
Meal 2	Kale chips	Black Bean Burger	Chicken Lollipops	Turkey Quesadilla	Pork Shoulder Skewers with Pineapple	Spaghetti Meatballs on Stick	Lamb Pie
Meal3	Sticky BBQ Honey Strips	Mediterranean Lamb Burgers	Potato Croquettes	Vegetable Fritters	Chicken Wings	Cheese Stuffed Turkey Meatballs	Balsamic Pork

112	Monday	Tuesday	Wednesday	Thursday	Friday	saturday	sunday
Meal 1	Turkey Meatloaf	Chicken Pie	Crispy Pork	Crispy Mongolian Beef	Plum Roast Lamb	Cheesy Zucchini boat	Cinnamon Sugar Churros
Meal 2	Teriyaki Beef Steak with Broccoli	Thai Lamb Stir Fry	Vegetable Spring rolls	Tropical Egg Rolls	Turkey Pattie with Avocado Salad	Chicken Sandwich	Pork Dumplings
Meal3	Thai Chicken Skewers	BBQ Pork Sandwich	Beef Kabobs	Classic Lamb Shanks	Veggie Stuffed Peppers	Chocolate Cake	Turkey Burgers

WEEK 113	Monday	Tuesday	Wednesday	Thursday	Friday	saturday	sunday
Meal 1	BBQ Pulled Pork with Coleslaw	Turkey Sausages	Almond Stuffed Chicken	Skirt Steak Fajitas Wraps	Roasted Lamb Leg	Tofu Satay	Chocolate Soufflé
Meal 2	Sweet Potato Jackets	Sticky BBQ Tofu	Herb Crusted Pork Ribs	Cranberry Turkey Wings	Sticky Lemon Drumsticks	Thai Beef Salad	Lamb Steak with Sweet Potatoes
Meal3	Chinese beef and Broccoli	Basil Lamb Cutlets	Vegetable Lasagna	Sweet and Sour Cauliflower Stir fry	Pork Steaks with Broccoli	Mexican Turkey Tacos	Tandoori Masala Chicken

WEEK 114	Monday	Tuesday	Wednesday	Thursday	Friday	saturday	sunday
Meal 1	Chicken Wings	Butter-Honey Glazed Turkey	Buttery Pork Chops	Teriyaki Beef Steak with Broccoli	Classic Lamb Shanks	Blooming Onion with Spicy dip	Chocolate Fudge Brownies
Meal 2	Cheesy Jalapenos	Coconut Cookies	Crispy Garlic Chicken with Lemon Dip	Pineapple Turkey Kabobs	BBQ Pulled Pork with Coleslaw	Beef chipotle	Lemon Herb Lamb Chops
Meal3	Lemon Herb Beef Roast	Thai Lamb Stir Fry	Eggplant Pizza	Assorted Donuts	Rotisserie Chicken	Lemon Garlic Turkey	Balsamic Pork

WEEK 115	Monday	Tuesday	Wednesday	Thursday	Friday	saturday	sunday
Meal 1	Beef Stuffed Capsicum	Lamb Pie	Vegan Burrito Bowl	Pineapple Bites	Mexican Chicken Wrap	Pistachio Stuffed Turkey Breast	Pork Medallions with Sour Cream
Meal 2	Pulled Turkey Sandwich	Pork Shoulder Skewers with Pineapple	Spaghetti Meatballs on Stick	Mediterranean Lamb Burgers	Potato Croquettes	Raisin Bread Pudding with Chocolate	BBQ Chicken Pizza
Meal3	Blueberry Cheesecake	Chicken Lollipops	Apricot Glazed Turkey Legs	Pork Quesadillas	Salted beef with Caramelized Onions	Sweet and Sour Lamb Ribs	Buffalo Cauliflower Wings

106

WEEK 116	Monday	Tuesday	Wednesday	Thursday	Friday	saturday	sunday
Meal 1	Crispy Coconut Pork Belly	Sticky BBQ Honey Strips	Kale chips	Classic Falafel	Chicken Nuggets	Turkey Quesadilla	Spicy Lamb Meatballs with Mango Salsa
Meal 2	Turkey Meatloaf	Walnut-Stuffed Lamb	Lemon Pork Ribs	Beef with Mix Vegetables	Vegetable Sushi	Black Bean Burger	Roasted Almond Chicken
Meal 3	Vegetable Fritters	Chicken Sandwich	Cheese Stuffed Turkey Meatballs	Turkish Kebabs with Tahini Sauce	Honey Mustard Pork Chops	Thai Beef Salad	Vegan Tacos

117	Monday	Tuesday	Wednesday	Thursday	Friday	saturday	sunday
Meal 1	Mexican Turkey Tacos	Lamb Steak with Sweet Potatoes	Chocolate Cake	Skirt Steak Fajitas Wraps	Herb Crusted Pork Ribs	Sticky Lemon Drumsticks	Veggie Stuffed Peppers
Meal 2	Chicken Pie	Tofu Satay	Turkey Burgers	Plum Roast Lamb	Cinnamon Sugar Churros	Crispy Mongolian Beef	Crispy Pork
Meal 3	Beef and Mushroom Meatloaf	BBQ Pork Sandwich	Almond Stuffed Chicken	Sweet Potato Jackets	Turkey Sausages	Crispy Cheesy Lamb Chops	Tropical Egg Rolls

WEEK 118	Monday	Tuesday	Wednesday	Thursday	Friday	saturday	sunday
Meal 1	Chocolate Soufflé	Chinese beef and Broccoli	Pork Steaks with Broccoli	Tandoori Masala Chicken	Basil Lamb Cutlets	Vegetable Lasagna	Turkey Pattie with Avocado Salad
Meal 2	Vegetable Spring rolls	Cranberry Turkey Wings	Sweet and Sour Cauliflower Stir fry	Beef Kabobs	Pork Dumplings	Thai Chicken Skewers	Classic Lamb Shanks
Meal 3	Chicken Wings	Roasted Lamb Leg	Cheesy Zucchini boat	Lemon Garlic Turkey	Sticky BBQ Tofu	Beef chipotle	Balsamic Pork

WEEK 119	Monday	Tuesday	Wednesday	Thursday	Friday	saturday	sunday
Meal 1	Lemon Herb Lamb Chops	Blooming Onion with Spicy dip	Butter-Honey Glazed Turkey	Chocolate Fudge Brownies	Crispy Garlic Chicken with Lemon Dip	Buttery Pork Chops	Teriyaki Beef Steak with Broccoli
Meal 2	Pork Medallions with Sour Cream	Beef Stuffed Capsicum	Mediterranean Lamb Burgers	Vegan Burrito Bowl	Pistachio Stuffed Turkey Breast	Pineapple Bites	Mexican Chicken Wrap
Meal 3	Classic Falafel	Chicken Nuggets	Crispy Coconut Pork Belly	Sticky BBQ Honey Strips	Spicy Lamb Meatballs with Mango Salsa	Kale chips	Turkey Quesadilla

WEEK 120	Monday	Tuesday	Wednesday	Thursday	Friday	saturday	sunday
Meal 1	Thai Lamb Stir Fry	Eggplant Pizza	BBQ Pulled Pork with Coleslaw	Lemon Herb Beef Roast	Pineapple Turkey Kabobs	Rotisserie Chicken	Assorted Donuts
Meal 2	BBQ Chicken Pizza	Blueberry Cheesecake	Lamb Pie	Buffalo Cauliflower Wings	Pork Shoulder Skewers with Pineapple	Spaghetti Meatballs on Stick	Pulled Turkey Sandwich

Meal 3 Beef with Mix Vegetables   Turkey Meatloaf   Roasted Almond Chicken   Vegetable Fritters   Walnut-Stuffed Lamb   Vegan Tacos   Lemon Pork Ribs

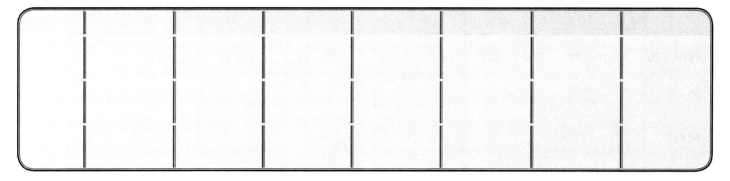

121	Monday	Tuesday	Wednesday	Thursday	Friday	saturday	sunday
Meal 1	Chicken Lollipops	Apricot Glazed Turkey Legs	Pork Quesadillas	Salted beef with Caramelized Onions	Sweet and Sour Lamb Ribs	Cheesy Jalapenos	Coconut Cookies
Meal 2	Veggie Stuffed Peppers	Chocolate Cake	Chicken Sandwich	Cheese Stuffed Turkey Meatballs	Honey Mustard Pork Chops	Thai Beef Salad	Turkish Kebabs with Tahini Sauce
Meal3	Beef chipotle	Basil Lamb Cutlets	Tofu Satay	Cinnamon Sugar Churros	Chicken Wings	Lemon Garlic Turkey	Pork Steaks with Broccoli

WEEK 122	Monday	Tuesday	Wednesday	Thursday	Friday	saturday	sunday
Meal 1	Herb Crusted Pork Ribs	Skirt Steak Fajitas Wraps	Potato Croquettes	Sticky Lemon Drumsticks	Mexican Turkey Tacos	Lamb Steak with Sweet Potatoes	Raisin Bread Pudding with Chocolate
Meal 2	Classic Lamb Shanks	Chocolate Soufflé	Pork Dumplings	Chinese beef and Broccoli	Vegetable Lasagna	Tandoori Masala Chicken	Turkey Pattie with Avocado Salad
Meal3	Thai Chicken Skewers	Cranberry Turkey Wings	Roasted Lamb Leg	Sweet and Sour Cauliflower Stir fry	Balsamic Pork	Beef Kabobs	Vegetable Spring rolls

WEEK 123	Monday	Tuesday	Wednesday	Thursday	Friday	saturday	sunday
Meal 1	Chicken Pie	Turkey Burgers	Crispy Pork	Crispy Mongolian Beef	Plum Roast Lamb	Vegetable Sushi	Black Bean Burger
Meal 2	Almond Stuffed Chicken	Turkey Sausages	BBQ Pork Sandwich	Beef and Mushroom Meatloaf	Crispy Cheesy Lamb Chops	Sweet Potato Jackets	Tropical Egg Rolls
Meal3	Crispy Garlic Chicken with Lemon Dip	Butter-Honey Glazed Turkey	Buttery Pork Chops	Teriyaki Beef Steak with Broccoli	Lemon Herb Lamb Chops	Cheesy Zucchini boat	Sticky BBQ Tofu

WEEK 124	Monday	Tuesday	Wednesday	Thursday	Friday	saturday	sunday
Meal 1	Pork Medallions with Sour Cream	Chocolate Fudge Brownies	Mediterranean Lamb Burgers	Mexican Chicken Wrap	Beef Stuffed Capsicum	Blooming Onion with Spicy dip	Turkey Quesadilla
Meal 2	Lemon Herb Beef Roast	Buffalo Cauliflower Wings	Pineapple Turkey Kabobs	Pork Shoulder Skewers with Pineapple	Blueberry Cheesecake	Thai Lamb Stir Fry	Rotisserie Chicken
Meal3	Cinnamon Sugar Churros	Sweet and Sour Lamb Ribs	Chicken Lollipops	Salted beef with Caramelized Onions	Tofu Satay	Apricot Glazed Turkey Legs	Honey Mustard Pork Chops

WEEK 125	Monday	Tuesday	Wednesday	Thursday	Friday	saturday	sunday
Meal 1	Pistachio Stuffed Turkey Breast	Sticky BBQ Honey Strips	Crispy Coconut Pork Belly	Chicken Nuggets	Spicy Lamb Meatballs with Mango Salsa	Vegan Burrito Bowl	Pineapple Bites
Meal 2	Eggplant Pizza	Assorted Donuts	Pulled Turkey Sandwich	Spaghetti Meatballs on Stick	Lemon Pork Ribs	Roasted Almond Chicken	Lamb Pie
Meal3	Chicken Sandwich	Turkish Kebabs with Tahini Sauce	Veggie Stuffed Peppers	Chocolate Cake	Cheese Stuffed Turkey Meatballs	Thai Beef Salad	Pork Steaks with Broccoli

WEEK 126	Monday	Tuesday	Wednesday	Thursday	Friday	saturday	sunday
Meal 1	Kale chips	Walnut-Stuffed Lamb	BBQ Pulled Pork with Coleslaw	BBQ Chicken Pizza	Classic Falafel	Turkey Meatloaf	Beef with Mix Vegetables
Meal 2	Lemon Garlic Turkey	Beef chipotle	Potato Croquettes	Basil Lamb Cutlets	Herb Crusted Pork Ribs	Chicken Wings	Raisin Bread Pudding with Chocolate
Meal 3	Crispy Garlic Chicken with Lemon Dip	Chocolate Soufflé	Butter-Honey Glazed Turkey	Teriyaki Beef Steak with Broccoli	Vegetable Lasagna	Classic Lamb Shanks	Buttery Pork Chops

WEEK 127	Monday	Tuesday	Wednesday	Thursday	Friday	saturday	sunday
Meal 1	Lamb Steak with Sweet Potatoes	Mexican Turkey Tacos	Vegetable Fritters	Pork Dumplings	Skirt Steak Fajitas Wraps	Vegan Tacos	Sticky Lemon Drumsticks
Meal 2	Cheesy Jalapenos	Chicken Pie	Plum Roast Lamb	Turkey Burgers	Coconut Cookies	Crispy Pork	Crispy Mongolian Beef
Meal 3	BBQ Pork Sandwich	Beef and Mushroom Meatloaf	Sweet Potato Jackets	Almond Stuffed Chicken	Crispy Cheesy Lamb Chops	Turkey Sausages	Tropical Egg Rolls

WEEK 128	Monday	Tuesday	Wednesday	Thursday	Friday	saturday	sunday
Meal 1	Pork Quesadillas	Vegetable Spring rolls	Tandoori Masala Chicken	Turkey Pattie with Avocado Salad	Sweet and Sour Cauliflower Stir fry	Chinese beef and Broccoli	Roasted Lamb Leg
Meal 2	Beef Kabobs	Lemon Herb Lamb Chops	Balsamic Pork	Vegetable Sushi	Thai Chicken Skewers	Cranberry Turkey Wings	Black Bean Burger
Meal 3	Turkey Quesadilla	Sticky BBQ Tofu	Beef Stuffed Capsicum	Mediterranean Lamb Burgers	Pork Medallions with Sour Cream	Cheesy Zucchini boat	Mexican Chicken Wrap

WEEK 129	Monday	Tuesday	Wednesday	Thursday	Friday	saturday	sunday
Meal 1	Rotisserie Chicken	Pineapple Turkey Kabobs	Chicken Nuggets	Pistachio Stuffed Turkey Breast	BBQ Chicken Pizza	Turkey Meatloaf	Blueberry Cheesecake
Meal 2	Crispy Coconut Pork Belly	Buffalo Cauliflower Wings	BBQ Pulled Pork with Coleslaw	Vegan Burrito Bowl	Pork Shoulder Skewers with Pineapple	Kale chips	Beef with Mix Vegetables
Meal 3	Classic Falafel	Spicy Lamb Meatballs with Mango Salsa	Pineapple Bites	Thai Lamb Stir Fry	Sticky BBQ Honey Strips	Lemon Herb Beef Roast	Walnut-Stuffed Lamb

WEEK 130	Monday	Tuesday	Wednesday	Thursday	Friday	saturday	sunday
Meal 1	Salted beef with Caramelized Onions	Apricot Glazed Turkey Legs	Cinnamon Sugar Churros	Honey Mustard Pork Chops	Chicken Lollipops	Tofu Satay	Sweet and Sour Lamb Ribs
Meal 2	Eggplant Pizza	Lamb Pie	Spaghetti Meatballs on Stick	Pulled Turkey Sandwich	Assorted Donuts	Lemon Pork Ribs	Roasted Almond Chicken
Meal 3	Buttery Pork Chops	Crispy Garlic Chicken with Lemon Dip	Vegetable Lasagna	Classic Lamb Shanks	Teriyaki Beef Steak with Broccoli	Butter-Honey Glazed Turkey	Chocolate Soufflé

WEEK 131	Monday	Tuesday	Wednesday	Thursday	Friday	saturday	sunday
Meal 1	Turkish Kebabs with Tahini Sauce	Chocolate Cake	Pork Steaks with Broccoli	Chicken Sandwich	Cheese Stuffed Turkey Meatballs	Veggie Stuffed Peppers	Thai Beef Salad
Meal 2	Potato Croquettes	Beef chipotle	Basil Lamb Cutlets	Raisin Bread Pudding with Chocolate	Herb Crusted Pork Ribs	Chicken Wings	Lemon Garlic Turkey
Meal3	Mexican Chicken Wrap	Turkey Quesadilla	Blooming Onion with Spicy dip	Beef Stuffed Capsicum	Mediterranean Lamb Burgers	Chocolate Fudge Brownies	Pork Medallions with Sour Cream

WEEK 132	Monday	Tuesday	Wednesday	Thursday	Friday	saturday	sunday
Meal 1	Vegetable Fritters	Mexican Turkey Tacos	Lamb Steak with Sweet Potatoes	Skirt Steak Fajitas Wraps	Sticky Lemon Drumsticks	Vegan Tacos	Pork Dumplings
Meal 2	Vegetable Sushi	Pork Quesadillas	Black Bean Burger	Turkey Pattie with Avocado Salad	Roasted Lamb Leg	Chinese beef and Broccoli	Tandoori Masala Chicken
Meal3	Beef Kabobs	Thai Chicken Skewers	Cheesy Zucchini boat	Balsamic Pork	Sticky BBQ Tofu	Cranberry Turkey Wings	Lemon Herb Lamb Chops

WEEK 133	Monday	Tuesday	Wednesday	Thursday	Friday	saturday	sunday
Meal 1	Chicken Pie	Turkey Burgers	Crispy Pork	Crispy Mongolian Beef	Plum Roast Lamb	Cheesy Jalapenos	Coconut Cookies
Meal 2	Crispy Cheesy Lamb Chops	Sweet Potato Jackets	Tropical Egg Rolls	Almond Stuffed Chicken	Turkey Sausages	BBQ Pork Sandwich	Beef and Mushroom Meatloaf
Meal3	Pistachio Stuffed Turkey Breast	Crispy Coconut Pork Belly	Sticky BBQ Honey Strips	Spicy Lamb Meatballs with Mango Salsa	Vegetable Spring rolls	Sweet and Sour Cauliflower Stir fry	Chicken Nuggets

WEEK 134	Monday	Tuesday	Wednesday	Thursday	Friday	saturday	sunday
Meal 1	Turkey Meatloaf	BBQ Pulled Pork with Coleslaw	BBQ Chicken Pizza	Beef with Mix Vegetables	Kale chips	Classic Falafel	Walnut-Stuffed Lamb
Meal 2	Eggplant Pizza	Assorted Donuts	Lamb Pie	Pulled Turkey Sandwich	Lemon Pork Ribs	Roasted Almond Chicken	Spaghetti Meatballs on Stick
Meal3	Herb Crusted Pork Ribs	Chicken Wings	Beef chipotle	Potato Croquettes	Raisin Bread Pudding with Chocolate	Basil Lamb Cutlets	Lemon Garlic Turkey

WEEK 135	Monday	Tuesday	Wednesday	Thursday	Friday	saturday	sunday
Meal 1	Pork Shoulder Skewers with Pineapple	Pineapple Turkey Kabobs	Buffalo Cauliflower Wings	Lemon Herb Beef Roast	Thai Lamb Stir Fry	Rotisserie Chicken	Blueberry Cheesecake
Meal 2	Classic Lamb Shanks	Crispy Garlic Chicken with Lemon Dip	Chocolate Soufflé	Buttery Pork Chops	Butter-Honey Glazed Turkey	Vegetable Lasagna	Teriyaki Beef Steak with Broccoli
Meal3	Mexican Turkey Tacos	Vegan Tacos	Skirt Steak Fajitas Wraps	Lamb Steak with Sweet Potatoes	Sticky Lemon Drumsticks	Vegetable Fritters	Pork Dumplings

WEEK 136	Monday	Tuesday	Wednesday	Thursday	Friday	saturday	sunday
Meal 1	Chicken Lollipops	Apricot Glazed Turkey Legs	Honey Mustard Pork Chops	Salted beef with Caramelized Onions	Sweet and Sour Lamb Ribs	Vegan Burrito Bowl	Pineapple Bites
Meal 2	Vegetable Sushi	Black Bean Burger	Chicken Sandwich	Turkey Quesadilla	Pork Steaks with Broccoli	Thai Beef Salad	Turkish Kebabs with Tahini Sauce
Meal3	Sticky BBQ Honey Strips	Spicy Lamb Meatballs with Mango Salsa	Cheesy Jalapenos	Coconut Cookies	Chicken Nuggets	Pistachio Stuffed Turkey Breast	Crispy Coconut Pork Belly

WEEK 137	Monday	Tuesday	Wednesday	Thursday	Friday	saturday	sunday
Meal 1	Cinnamon Sugar Churros	Tofu Satay	Pork Medallions with Sour Cream	Mexican Chicken Wrap	Cheese Stuffed Turkey Meatballs	Beef Stuffed Capsicum	Mediterranean Lamb Burgers
Meal 2	Turkey Pattie with Avocado Salad	Chinese beef and Broccoli	Roasted Lamb Leg	Chocolate Fudge Brownies	Blooming Onion with Spicy dip	Pork Quesadillas	Thai Chicken Skewers
Meal3	Vegetable Spring rolls	BBQ Pork Sandwich	Chicken Pie	Turkey Burgers	Beef and Mushroom Meatloaf	Crispy Cheesy Lamb Chops	Sweet and Sour Cauliflower Stir fry

WEEK 138	Monday	Tuesday	Wednesday	Thursday	Friday	saturday	sunday
Meal 1	Beef Kabobs	Lemon Herb Lamb Chops	Veggie Stuffed Peppers	Chocolate Cake	Tandoori Masala Chicken	Cranberry Turkey Wings	Balsamic Pork
Meal 2	Turkey Sausages	Crispy Pork	Crispy Mongolian Beef	Plum Roast Lamb	Cheesy Zucchini boat	Sticky BBQ Tofu	Almond Stuffed Chicken
Meal3	Tropical Egg Rolls	BBQ Chicken Pizza	Turkey Meatloaf	BBQ Pulled Pork with Coleslaw	Beef with Mix Vegetables	Walnut-Stuffed Lamb	Sweet Potato Jackets

WEEK 139	Monday	Tuesday	Wednesday	Thursday	Friday	saturday	sunday
Meal 1	Pulled Turkey Sandwich	Lemon Pork Ribs	Roasted Almond Chicken	Spaghetti Meatballs on Stick	Lamb Pie	Classic Falafel	Kale chips
Meal 2	Blueberry Cheesecake	Buffalo Cauliflower Wings	Pineapple Turkey Kabobs	Pork Shoulder Skewers with Pineapple	Rotisserie Chicken	Lemon Herb Beef Roast	Thai Lamb Stir Fry
Meal3	Salted beef with Caramelized Onion	Sweet and Sour Lamb Ribs	Pineapple Bites	Vegan Burrito Bowl	Apricot Glazed Turkey Legs	Honey Mustard Pork Chops	Chicken Lollipops

WEEK 140	Monday	Tuesday	Wednesday	Thursday	Friday	saturday	sunday
Meal 1	Chicken Wings	Lemon Garlic Turkey	Herb Crusted Pork Ribs	Beef chipotle	Basil Lamb Cutlets	Eggplant Pizza	Assorted Donuts
Meal 2	Vegetable Lasagna	Chocolate Soufflé	Crispy Garlic Chicken with Lemon Dip	Butter-Honey Glazed Turkey	Buttery Pork Chops	Teriyaki Beef Steak with Broccoli	Classic Lamb Shanks
Meal3	Sticky BBQ Honey Strips	Spicy Lamb Meatballs with Mango Salsa	Vegetable Sushi	Black Bean Burger	Chicken Nuggets	Pistachio Stuffed Turkey Breast	Crispy Coconut Pork Belly

110

141	Monday	Tuesday	Wednesday	Thursday	Friday	saturday	sunday
Meal 1	Raisin Bread Pudding with Chocolate	Pork Dumplings	Potato Croquettes	Mexican Turkey Tacos	Skirt Steak Fajitas Wraps	Sticky Lemon Drumsticks	Lamb Steak with Sweet Potatoes
Meal 2	Chicken Sandwich	Turkish Kebabs with Tahini Sauce	Cinnamon Sugar Churros	Pork Steaks with Broccoli	Tofu Satay	Turkey Quesadilla	Thai Beef Salad
Meal 3	Turkey Meatloaf	Beef with Mix Vegetables	BBQ Chicken Pizza	Walnut-Stuffed Lamb	Chocolate Cake	BBQ Pulled Pork with Coleslaw	Veggie Stuffed Peppers

WEEK 142	Monday	Tuesday	Wednesday	Thursday	Friday	saturday	sunday
Meal 1	Mediterranean Lamb Burgers	Vegan Tacos	Vegetable Fritters	Mexican Chicken Wrap	Cheese Stuffed Turkey Meatballs	Pork Medallions with Sour Cream	Beef Stuffed Capsicum
Meal 2	Balsamic Pork	Beef Kabobs	Lemon Herb Lamb Chops	Blooming Onion with Spicy dip	Chocolate Fudge Brownies	Tandoori Masala Chicken	Cranberry Turkey Wings
Meal 3	Almond Stuffed Chicken	Turkey Sausages	Crispy Pork	Crispy Mongolian Beef	Plum Roast Lamb	Sweet Potato Jackets	Tropical Egg Rolls

WEEK 143	Monday	Tuesday	Wednesday	Thursday	Friday	saturday	sunday
Meal 1	Pork Quesadillas	Cheesy Jalapenos	Thai Chicken Skewers	Turkey Pattie with Avocado Salad	Coconut Cookies	Roasted Lamb Leg	Chinese beef and Broccoli
Meal 2	Crispy Cheesy Lamb Chops	Beef and Mushroom Meatloaf	BBQ Pork Sandwich	Vegetable Spring rolls	Chicken Pie	Turkey Burgers	Sweet and Sour Cauliflower Stir fry
Meal 3	Pulled Turkey Sandwich	Sticky BBQ Tofu	Lamb Pie	Spaghetti Meatballs on Stick	Lemon Pork Ribs	Cheesy Zucchini boat	Roasted Almond Chicken

CPSIA information can be obtained
at www.ICGtesting.com
Printed in the USA
LVHW061807010621
689061LV00004B/708